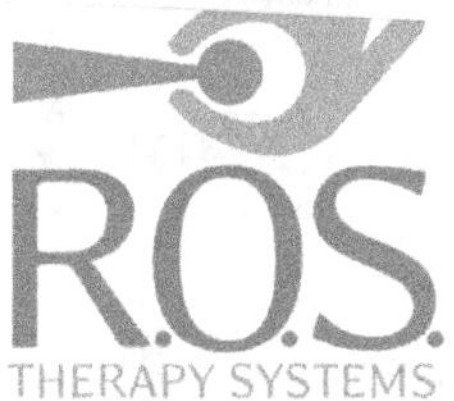

R.O.S. Therapy Systems Presents:

Caregiver Activity Lesson Plans

December and Christmas Activities

Word Scramble

Code Breakers

Word Search

Crossword

Trivia

How Much Do You Know About?

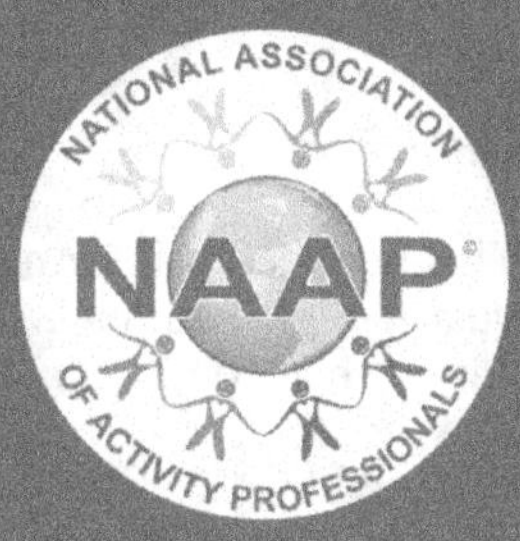

Scott Silknitter

VOLUME 4

Caregiver Activity Lesson Plans

How Much Do You Know About December and Christmas

This edition of the *Caregiver Activity Lesson Plans* features some of the favorite activities of leading Activity Professionals from around the United States. Activity Professionals are the quality of life experts that focus on the social side of long-term care and design individual programs for every resident, client or participant they work with. We have adapted those activities to make a booklet of one-to-one activities that can be used by any caregiver in any setting.

About NAAP

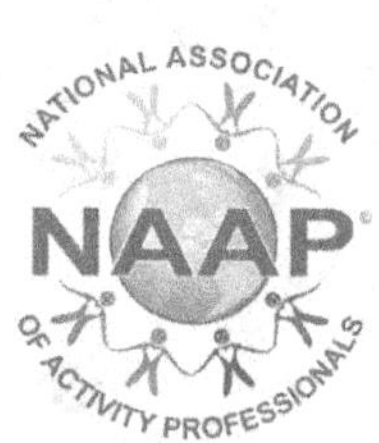

Since 1981, the National Association of Activity Professionals (NAAP) has led the way for activities for residents in long-term care settings. Whether it is lobbying for and setting standards, educating members and the general public or promoting quality of life initiatives for those in any institutional setting, NAAP has been the driving force behind person-centered and person-appropriate social care.

About R.O.S. Therapy Systems

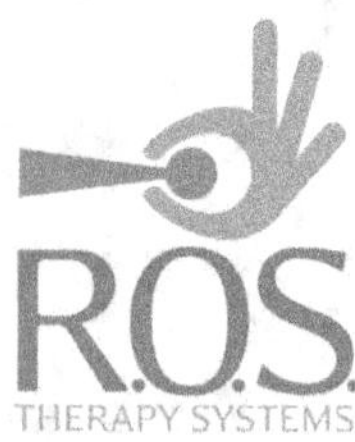

R.O.S. Therapy Systems began as a backyard project to help one family with their quality of life during a 25-year fight with Parkinson's and dementia. The company has grown into a trusted partner for Family Caregivers, Home Care Agencies, Adult Day Centers, Assisted Living Facilities and Skilled Nursing Facilities.

ISBN 978-1518604270

Disclaimer

This book is for informational and entertainment purposes only. All activities should be conducted under the supervision of a qualified professional, such as a Home Care Certified individual. At no time should a senior or other acting participant be left alone when conducting the activities listed in this book.

Published by
R.O.S. Therapy Systems, L.L.C.
Greensboro, NC
888-352-9788
www.ROSTherapySystems.com

How to use an Activity Lesson Plan:

An Activity Lesson Plan should be ever-changing. It is meant to be written on and to note the changes you may have made from the original plan so that the next person working with the participant can follow your modifications with the goal of recreating positive experiences.

Date: Document the date the activity is used with the participant

Activity Name: Name of the activity being performed

Objective: To provide meaningful, purposeful activities that will engage

Materials: Suggested materials and resources to use with this activity

Prerequisite Skills: Skills and abilities a person should possess for this activity

Activity Outline: Step-by-step instructions to complete the activity

Evaluation: A thorough evaluation is the most important part of the Lesson Plan. When conducting an activity with the participant, record any verbal cues, assistance, or modifications to incorporate into the activity. It is also helpful to include the participants response to the program.

Note programs that are successful at distracting or eliminating a negative behavior (diversion activities). Encourage family members and caregivers to use the evaluation section and also leave tips. Don't waste time recreating the wheel of knowledge. Pass on the information so everyone presents the activity in the same way with the same modifications and cueing, in order to achieve the same positive outcomes.

**** A leader must be present at all times when conducting the activities contained in this book.**

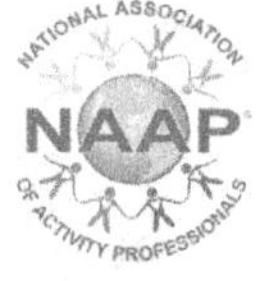

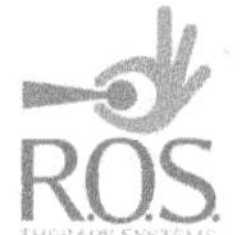

Every person has his or her own unique physical and cognitive abilities and needs. How that person responds to an activity will dictate how the leader will continue to modify or adapt an Activity Lesson Plan to meet an individual participants needs and abilities – now and in the future.

It is up to the leader to determine modifications to any Activity Lesson Plan so an activity is person-centered and person-appropriate. The following is an example of modifying an activity:

Butterfly Craft

You know that the participant loves butterflies. You decide to use an Activity Lesson Plan based on a butterfly craft. Depending on the participants physical and cognitive level, you will determine what adjustments have to be made. Here are examples of four functional levels and how your butterfly activity may be modified:

- Level 1: Coffee Filter Butterfly Craft: Take a coffee filter and paint it with watercolor paint. When it dries, pinch the center together and tie a pipe cleaner around the center in the shape of a butterfly body. Make two antennas out of the pipe cleaners.
- Level 2: Color pictures of butterflies
- Level 3: Look at the pictures and discuss butterflies together
- Level 4: The leader shows pictures of butterflies to the participant

To ensure the participant reaps the benefits of being engaged, please adapt any and all activities to the participants functional level.

The leader should read all step-by-step directions of an Activity Outline before beginning an activity with a participant. The step-by-step directions are general guidelines for the leader to use, and potentially modify, in order to help the participant successfully engage in the chosen activity.

Thank you for using this edition of Caregiver Activity Lesson Plans

R.O.S. Therapy Systems offers several *Caregiver Activity Lesson Plan* books. We have amassed hundreds of Activity Lesson Plans so there is something for everyone:

- Craft Activities
- Holiday Activities
- Activities for Men
- Music Activities
- Gardening Activities
- Games
- Baking Activities
- Verbal Communication Skills Activities
- Outdoor Activities
- Science Activities
- Art Activities
- Computer Activities

Please check www.ROSTherapySystems.com or www.therosstore.com to see a complete list of available *Caregiver Activity Lesson Plans* books. With new books being published regularly, please check back often.

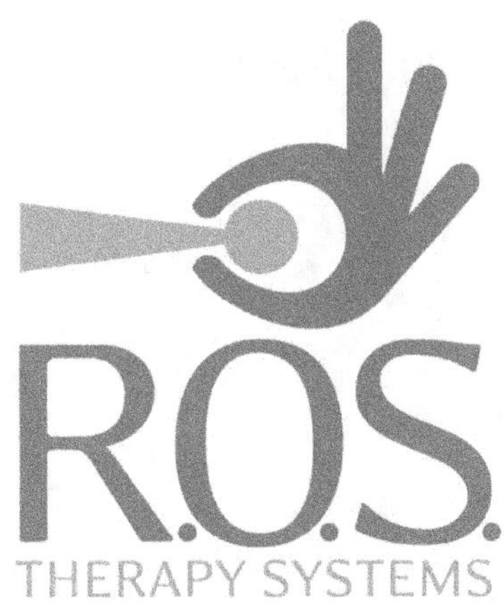

If we can help in any other way, please contact us directly at 888-352-9788

Caregiver Activity Lesson Plans How Much Do You Know About: December and Christmas

Table of Contents

Caregiver Activity Lesson Plans
How Much Do You Know About:
December and Christmas

Table of Contents

Activity Lesson Plans

December and Christmas Trivia

December and Christmas Trivia

- The following pages contain basic templates that can be used by anyone. The leader must allow for the participant to be successful.
- The leader should read all step-by-step directions of an Activity Outline before beginning an activity with a participant. The step-by-step directions are general guidelines for the leader/caregiver to use and potentially modify in order to help the participant successfully engage in the chosen activity.
- The leader must always be present when engaging the participant in an activity.
- The leader must take all necessary and reasonable precautions to ensure the safety of the participant.
- The leader should have necessary materials ready and prepared prior to the beginning of the activity.
- To ensure that the participant reaps the benefits of being engaged, please adapt any and all activities to the participants functional level.

Program Name: December Trivia **Date:** ____________

Leader: ______________________________ **Time:** ____________

Objective:

- Stimulate cognitive functioning
- Increase self-worth and improve self-esteem
- Increase socialization
- Foster friendship, laughter and closeness
- Provide a sense of accomplishment
- Stimulate memory
- Have some fun!

Materials:

- Flat surface for participant to write on
- Templates on the following pages provided
- Pen, pencil or high lighter

Note: If a participant is in a bed, recliner or wheelchair, consider using the R.O.S. Multi-Purpose Board Insert and the R.O.S. Legacy™ System Console available at R.O.S. Therapy Systems (www.therosstore.com) as an option for a flat surface to allow the participant the opportunity to fully engage in this activity.

Prerequisite Skills:

Every person has his or her own unique physical/cognitive abilities and needs. How a participant responds to an activity will dictate how the caregiver will modify or adapt a Lesson Plan to meet individual client needs and abilities – now and in the future.

Program Name: December Trivia **Date:** ____________

Leader: ______________________________ **Time:** ____________

Activity Outline:

The leader explains to the participant that they will be playing a trivia game.

1. Use the following templates to enjoy trivia based on topics of interest.

Option 1: Based on the participants abilities, the participant completes the activity on their own.

Option 2: Based on the participants abilities, the leader assists with finding answers.

Option 3: Based on the participants abilities, the leader and the participant have a discussion based on words and topics included in this activity.

Evaluation:

December Trivia 1

1. What month of the year is December?

   ____

2. What does the Latin root word "decem" mean?

   ____

3. What are the major holidays in December?

   ____

4. What do people spend a lot of time doing in December?

   ____

5. In what season does December fall?

   ____

6. What special event happens on about December 20?

   ____

7. How many days are in December?

   ____

8. North American December is cold and wintry. What is it like in South America?

   ____

December Trivia 1

9. What happened on December 7, 1941?

____

10. Who called December 7, 1941 “a day which will live in infamy”?

____

11. British countries celebrate what holiday on December 26?

____

12. What days are Kwanzaa celebrated?

____

13. What plants are the often seen in December?

____

14. What zodiac signs are found in December?

____

15. What is December’s birthstone?

____

16. What are the 4 weeks before Christmas called in the Christian year?

____

December Trivia 1

17. How do you get mistletoe out of a tree?

____

18. What culture's calendar began in March, making December the 10th month?

____

19. What did the Wright brothers do on December 17, 1903?

____

20. Prize named after Swedish philanthropist awarded every December?

____

December Trivia 2

1. What is the last day of the year?

    ____

2. What might fall from the sky in December?

    ____

3. Whose feast day is December 6?

    ____

4. Who abdicated the English throne in December?

    ____

5. Who landed on Plymouth Rock in December 1620?

    ____

6. What ship serves as the Pearl Harbor memorial?

    ____

7. Who conceded one of the closest presidential elections in December 2000?

    ____

8. What celestial object was observed by Sir Edmund Halley on 12/25/1758?

    ____

December Trivia 2

9. What is December's birth flower?

 ____

10. What are people decking in December, and with what?

 ____

11. What are released in December with hopes for a blockbuster season?

 ____

12. What state was first to ratify the Constitution, 12/7/1777?

 ____

13. What kind of farm might you visit in December?

 ____

14. What do people bake a lot of in December?

 ____

15. What kind of edible house would you build in December?

 ____

16. If you saw a lot of short people running around in December, who might they be?

 ____

December Trivia 2

17. What do Italians traditionally serve on Christmas Eve?

    ____

18. How do you get to grandmother's house, in the song?

    ____

19. Why should you better watch out & better not cry?

    ____

20. Who introduced the first electric Christmas lights in December 1882?

    ____

December Trivia 1

(answers)

1. 12th
2. Ten
3. Christmas, New Year's Eve, Hanukkah (usually), Kwanzaa
4. Shopping
5. Winter
6. Winter solstice – longest night/shortest day, 1st day of winter
7. 31
8. Hot & summery
9. Pearl Harbor bombing
10. FDR
11. Boxing Day
12. Dec 26-Jan 1
13. Holly, poinsettia
14. Sagittarius (thru Dec 21), Capricorn (Dec 22-31)
15. Turquoise
16. Advent
17. Shoot it
18. Romans
19. Took their first flight – Kitty Hawk, NC
20. Nobel

December Trivia 2
(answers)

1. December 31
2. Snow
3. St. Nicholas
4. Edward VIII (Duke of Windsor)
5. Pilgrims
6. USS Arizona
7. Al Gore
8. Halley's comet
9. Narcissus
10. Halls with boughs of holly
11. Movies
12. Delaware
13. Christmas tree farm
14. Cookies
15. Gingerbread
16. Santa's elves
17. Fish – Feast of 7 fishes, 7-course fish meal
18. Over the river & through the woods
19. Santa Claus is coming to town
20. Thomas Edison

Christmas Trivia 1

1. What date is Christmas celebrated?

   ____

2. What is the night before Christmas called?

   ____

3. What jolly old man brings presents?

   ____

4. What color is Santa's suit?

   ____

5. What do people exchange at Christmas?

   ____

6. What do people send in the mail to each other at Christmas?

   ____

7. What do children hang on Christmas Eve?

   ____

8. What does Santa ride in?

   ____

Christmas Trivia 1

9. Who pulls Santa's sleigh?

 ____

10. How many reindeer does Santa have?

 ____

11. What are their names?

 ____

12. Which reindeer has a red nose?

 ____

13. Where does Santa live?

 ____

14. Who makes Santa's toys?

 ____

15. What are considered the two main Christmas colors?

 ____

16. What do people put in their houses to celebrate the Christmas season?

 ____

Christmas Trivia 1

17. What greeting do people use with each other?

    ____

18. What do Carolers do?

    ____

19. What do people hang on their front door at Christmas?

    ____

20. What does Santa Claus say?

    ____

Christmas Trivia 2

1. What do people sing at Christmas?

   ____

2. What did people put in Christmas trees before there were lights?

   ____

3. Whose birth does Christmas celebrate?

   ____

4. What is roasting on an open fire?

   ____

5. Traditional Christmas drink?

   ____

6. Traditional Christmas Wine?

   ____

7. A Christmas drink for the kids?

   ____

8. A favorite main dish for Christmas dinner?

   ____

Christmas Trivia 2

9. A fun and fruity holiday food?

____

10. What decoration do people put on their homes for the season?

____

11. What kind of Christmas was Bing Crosby dreaming of?

____

12. What famous poem was written about Christmas?

____

13. Who did Ebenezer Scrooge see?

____

14. What Dr. Seuss character stole Christmas?

____

15. Who wore a magic hat that brought him to life?

____

16. What famous Christmas movie starred Jimmy Stewart and Donna Reed?

____

Christmas Trivia 2

17. On what New York street did a miracle happen?

    ____

18. How many days of Christmas are there?

    ____

19. Who was seen kissing Santa Claus?

    ____

20. What is another name for Santa Claus?

    ____

Christmas Trivia 1
(answers)

1. December 25
2. Christmas Eve
3. Santa Claus
4. Red
5. Presents or gifts
6. Christmas cards
7. Stockings
8. Sleigh
9. Reindeer
10. 8
11. Dasher, Dancer, Prancer, Vixen, Comet, Cupid, Donner, Blitzen
12. Rudolph
13. North Pole
14. Elves
15. Red and green
16. Christmas trees
17. Merry Christmas!
18. Sing Christmas Carols
19. Wreath
20. "Ho ho ho"

Christmas Trivia 2
(answers)

1. Carols
2. Candles
3. Jesus
4. Chestnuts
5. Eggnog
6. Mulled
7. Hot Cocoa
8. Turkey
9. Fruitcake
10. Christmas Lights
11. White Christmas
12. "Twas The Night Before Christmas"
13. Ghosts of Christmas Past/Present/Future
14. The Grinch
15. Frosty the Snowman
16. "It's a Wonderful Life"
17. 34th Street "Miracle on 34th Street"
18. Twelve
19. Mommy
20. Father Christmas

Activity Lesson Plans

December and Christmas Word Scramble

December and Christmas Word Scramble

- The following pages contain basic templates that can be used by anyone. The leader must allow for the participant to be successful.
- The leader should read all step-by-step directions of an Activity Outline before beginning an activity with a participant. The step-by-step directions are general guidelines for the leader/caregiver to use and potentially modify in order to help the participant successfully engage in the chosen activity.
- The leader must always be present when engaging the participant in an activity.
- The leader must take all necessary and reasonable precautions to ensure the safety of the participant.
- The leader should have necessary materials ready and prepared prior to the beginning of the activity.
- To ensure that the participant reaps the benefits of being engaged, please adapt any and all activities to the participants functional level.

Program Name: December Word Scramble **Date:** ____________

Leader: ________________________________ **Time:** ____________

Objective:

- Stimulate cognitive functioning
- Increase self-worth and improve self-esteem
- Increase socialization
- Foster friendship, laughter and closeness
- Provide a sense of accomplishment
- Stimulate memory
- Have some fun!

Materials:

- Flat surface for participant to write on
- Templates on the following pages provided
- Pen, pencil or high lighter

Note: If a participant is in a bed, recliner or wheelchair, consider using the R.O.S. Multi-Purpose Board Insert and the R.O.S. Legacy™ System Console available at R.O.S. Therapy Systems (www.therosstore.com) as an option for a flat surface to allow the participant the opportunity to fully engage in this activity.

Prerequisite Skills:

Every person has his or her own unique physical/cognitive abilities and needs. How a participant responds to an activity will dictate how the caregiver will modify or adapt a Lesson Plan to meet individual client needs and abilities – now and in the future.

Program Name: December Word Scramble **Date:** ____________

Leader: ________________________________ **Time:** ____________

Activity Outline:

The leader explains to the participant that they will be working on a word scramble puzzle.

1. Use the following templates to enjoy a word scramble based on topics of interest.

Option 1: Based on the participants abilities, the participant completes the activity on their own.

Option 2: Based on the participants abilities, the leader assists with finding answers.

Option 3: Based on the participants abilities, the leader and the participant have a discussion based on words and topics included in this activity.

Evaluation:

December Terms 1 - Scramble

1. OESR _ _ _ _
2. NWE SRAEY EVE _ _ _   _ _ _ _ _   _ _ _
3. EATWHR _ _ _ _ _ _
4. MTOIELEST _ _ _ _ _ _ _ _ _
5. CSORELAR _ _ _ _ _ _ _ _
6. TINMEDIRW _ _ _ _ _ _ _ _ _
7. ZNCROI _ _ _ _ _ _
8. PTTEIAONSI _ _ _ _ _ _ _ _ _ _
9. AZANWKA _ _ _ _ _ _ _
10. WHISIAL _ _ _ _ _ _ _

December Terms 2 - Scramble

1. HCGPEANAM _ _ _ _ _ _ _ _ _
2. IMAMNAL _ _ _ _ _ _ _
3. RELWADEA _ _ _ _ _ _ _ _
4. ASSIWAL _ _ _ _ _ _ _
5. HWGTEI _ _ _ _ _ _
6. CANYD NACE _ _ _ _ _   _ _ _ _
7. EBBLUB GSLHTI _ _ _ _ _ _   _ _ _ _ _ _
8. GNRGBRDEIEA _ _ _ _ _ _ _ _ _ _ _
9. NLBOE _ _ _ _ _
10. LOYHL _ _ _ _ _

December Terms 3 - Scramble

1. YEUL LGO _ _ _ _   _ _ _
2. WONDISR _ _ _ _ _ _ _
3. TOPASTEO _ _ _ _ _ _ _ _
4. RWNIET _ _ _ _ _ _
5. CEDEM _ _ _ _ _
6. INGBXO ADY _ _ _ _ _ _   _ _ _
7. RLEDEID _ _ _ _ _ _ _
8. IYV _ _ _
9. YMHHEPRU RTOGAB _ _ _ _ _ _ _ _   _ _ _ _ _ _
10. TNAAS CUSLA _ _ _ _ _   _ _ _ _ _

December Terms 4 - Scramble

1. LWSAKFONE _ _ _ _ _ _ _ _ _
2. NOLBE _ _ _ _ _
3. DLCO _ _ _ _
4. AITSARIUGTS _ _ _ _ _ _ _ _ _ _ _
5. AELPR ORARBH _ _ _ _ _   _ _ _ _ _ _
6. WHTAC TINGH _ _ _ _ _   _ _ _ _ _
7. RETAFH ETIM _ _ _ _ _ _   _ _ _ _
8. NHCKAUHA _ _ _ _ _ _ _ _
9. TS HEPENTS _ _   _ _ _ _ _ _ _
10. NSSIURACS _ _ _ _ _ _ _ _ _

Holiday: Christmas Terms 1 - Scramble

1. ELEVS _ _ _ _ _

2. SACSRMITH EEV _ _ _ _ _ _ _ _ _   _ _ _

3. SNAAT ULASC _ _ _ _ _   _ _ _ _ _

4. EUSSJ _ _ _ _ _

5. THEEEBMLH _ _ _ _ _ _ _ _ _

6. JELYL _ _ _ _ _

7. EISW ENM _ _ _ _   _ _ _

8. EERHPDHSS _ _ _ _ _ _ _ _ _

9. BECEEMDR _ _ _ _ _ _ _ _

10. AREGMN _ _ _ _ _ _

Holiday: Christmas Terms 2 - Scramble

1. IGELHS _ _ _ _ _ _
2. CORSEOG _ _ _ _ _ _ _
3. ESNINRKNCAEF _ _ _ _ _ _ _ _ _ _ _ _
4. A SIAHCRTMS CAORL _   _ _ _ _ _ _ _ _ _   _ _ _ _ _
5. OGLD RSIGN _ _ _ _   _ _ _ _ _
6. EIWTH ARHICTSMS _ _ _ _ _   _ _ _ _ _ _ _ _ _
7. NGSEAL _ _ _ _ _ _
8. INGHRC _ _ _ _ _ _
9. URPHOLD _ _ _ _ _ _ _
10. LVTEEW _ _ _ _ _ _

Holiday: Christmas Terms 3 - Scramble

1. NOGXIB YDA _ _ _ _ _ _ _   _ _ _
2. YMINEHC _ _ _ _ _ _ _
3. MYMOM _ _ _ _ _
4. TNHOR PEOL _ _ _ _ _   _ _ _ _
5. ISCNKGOT _ _ _ _ _ _ _ _
6. SRPNETE _ _ _ _ _ _ _
7. SLOETITME _ _ _ _ _ _ _ _ _
8. FRTOSY _ _ _ _ _ _
9. UORNFWLDE _ _ _ _ _ _ _ _ _
10. AHTRMISCS ERTE _ _ _ _ _ _ _ _ _   _ _ _ _

Holiday: Christmas Terms 4 - Scramble

1. LLOYJ _ _ _ _ _
2. LSNTIE GNHIT _ _ _ _ _ _   _ _ _ _ _
3. ACLRMIE _ _ _ _ _ _ _
4. GIAVRNII _ _ _ _ _ _ _ _
5. NLACEDS _ _ _ _ _ _ _
6. VATNDE _ _ _ _ _ _
7. ENTLZBI _ _ _ _ _ _ _
8. LSEBL _ _ _ _ _
9. TS ICNSLOAH _ _   _ _ _ _ _ _ _ _
10. LASOCR _ _ _ _ _ _

December Terms 1 - Scramble

1. OESR — R o s e
2. NWE SRAEY EVE — N e w Y e a r s E v e
3. EATWHR — W r e a t h
4. MTOIELEST — M i s t l e t o e
5. CSORELAR — C a r o l e r s
6. TINMEDIRW — M i d w i n t e r
7. ZNCROI — Z i r c o n
8. PTTEIAONSI — P o i n s e t t i a
9. AZANWKA — K w a n z a a
10. WHISIAL — S w a h i l i

December Terms 2 - Scramble

1. HCGPEANAM — C h a m p a g n e
2. IMAMNAL — M a i l m a n
3. RELWADEA — D e l a w a r e
4. ASSIWAL — W a s s a i l
5. HWGTEI — W e i g h t
6. CANYD NACE — C a n d y C a n e
7. EBBLUB GSLHTI — B u b b l e L i g h t s
8. GNRGBRDEIEA — G i n g e r b r e a d
9. NLBOE — N o b e l
10. LOYHL — H o l l y

December Terms 3 - Scramble

1. YEUL LGO	Yule Log
2. WONDISR	Windsor
3. TOPASTEO	Potatoes
4. RWNIET	Winter
5. CEDEM	Decem
6. INGBXO ADY	Boxing Day
7. RLEDEID	Dreidel
8. IYV	Ivy
9. YMHHEPRU RTOGAB	Humphrey Bogart
10. TNAAS CUSLA	Santa Claus

December Terms 4 - Scramble

1. LWSAKFONE	Snowflake
2. NOLBE	Nobel
3. DLCO	Cold
4. AITSARIUGTS	Sagittarius
5. AELPR ORARBH	Pearl Harbor
6. WHTAC TINGH	Watch Night
7. RETAFH ETIM	Father Time
8. NHCKAUHA	Chanukah
9. TS HEPENTS	St Stephen
10. NSSIURACS	Narcissus

Holiday: Christmas Terms 1 - Scramble

1. ELEVS	E l v e s
2. SACSRMITH EEV	C h r i s t m a s E v e
3. SNAAT ULASC	S a n t a C l a u s
4. EUSSJ	J e s u s
5. THEEEBMLH	B e t h l e h e m
6. JELYL	J e l l y
7. EISW ENM	W i s e M e n
8. EERHPDHSS	S h e p h e r d s
9. BECEEMDR	D e c e m b e r
10. AREGMN	M a n g e r

Holiday: Christmas Terms 2 - Scramble

1. IGELHS	Sleigh
2. CORSEOG	Scrooge
3. ESNINRKNCAEF	Frankincense
4. A SIAHCRTMS CAORL	A Christmas Carol
5. OGLD RSIGN	Gold Rings
6. EIWTH ARHICTSMS	White Christmas
7. NGSEAL	Angels
8. INGHRC	Grinch
9. URPHOLD	Rudolph
10. LVTEEW	Twelve

Holiday: Christmas Terms 3 - Scramble

1. NOGXIB YDA	Boxing Day
2. YMINEHC	Chimney
3. MYMOM	Mommy
4. TNHOR PEOL	North Pole
5. ISCNKGOT	Stocking
6. SRPNETE	Present
7. SLOETITME	Mistletoe
8. FRTOSY	Frosty
9. UORNFWLDE	Wonderful
10. AHTRMISCS ERTE	Christmas Tree

Holiday: Christmas Terms 4 - Scramble

1. LLOYJ	J o l l y
2. LSNTIE GNHIT	S i l e n t N i g h t
3. ACLRMIE	M i r a c l e
4. GIAVRNII	V i r g i n i a
5. NLACEDS	C a n d l e s
6. VATNDE	A d v e n t
7. ENTLZBI	B l i t z e n
8. LSEBL	B e l l s
9. TS ICNSLOAH	S t N i c h o l a s
10. LASOCR	C a r o l s

Activity Lesson Plans

December and Christmas Word Search

December and Christmas Word Search

- The following pages contain basic templates that can be used by anyone. The leader must allow for the participant to be successful.
- The leader should read all step-by-step directions of an Activity Outline before beginning an activity with a participant. The step-by-step directions are general guidelines for the leader/ caregiver to use and potentially modify in order to help the participant successfully engage in the chosen activity.
- The leader must always be present when engaging the participant in an activity.
- The leader must take all necessary and reasonable precautions to ensure the safety of the participant.
- The leader should have necessary materials ready and prepared prior to the beginning of the activity.
- To ensure that the participant reaps the benefits of being engaged, please adapt any and all activities to the participants functional level.

Program Name: December Word Search **Date:** ____________

Leader: ______________________________ **Time:** ____________

Objective:

- Stimulate cognitive functioning
- Increase self-worth and improve self-esteem
- Increase socialization
- Foster friendship, laughter and closeness
- Provide a sense of accomplishment
- Stimulate memory
- Have some fun!

Materials:

- Flat surface for participant to write on
- Templates on the following pages provided
- Pen, pencil or high lighter

Note: If a participant is in a bed, recliner or wheelchair, consider using the R.O.S. Multi-Purpose Board Insert and the R.O.S. Legacy™ System Console available at R.O.S. Therapy Systems (www.therosstore.com) as an option for a flat surface to allow the participant the opportunity to fully engage in this activity.

Prerequisite Skills:

Every person has his or her own unique physical/cognitive abilities and needs. How a participant responds to an activity will dictate how the caregiver will modify or adapt a Lesson Plan to meet individual client needs and abilities – now and in the future.

Program Name: December Word Search **Date:** ____________

Leader: ______________________________ **Time:** ____________

Activity Outline:

The leader explains to the participant that they will be working on a Word Search puzzle.

1. Use the following templates to enjoy Word Search based on topics of interest.

Option 1: Based on the participants abilities, the participant completes the activity on their own.

Option 2: Based on the participants abilities, the leader assists with finding answers.

Option 3: Based on the participants abilities, the leader and participant have a discussion based on words and topics included in this activity.

Evaluation:

December Terms 1 - Wordsearch

```
G Y R P B C I R Z Y U V S D Z A X
R O S E H Z W U M K W A N Z A A R
R S X C X N E W Y E A R S E V E Q
R O M D T D Y F H A S W A H I L I
R E I P G H Y Y E K A T W N T Q G
P I S Y F P I M A I F E I S H J F
T O T S M V S B E I K Z N T N G C
X I L I Z M L D S F K B I V D E D
G T E C T I O U J Z X M K R P D J
F C T A O C H F U V W M I M C T N
K N O R I C Y E P M U C B H Y O P
O Z E O J G U H G V F H N U A N N
C Y V L P O I N S E T T I A T S W
Z U J E Z D O X M I D W I N T E R
H B U R F P G W P J A C R H K K S
Q Q G S D W R E A T H J R D S J P
L I L Y Y A F P A Q D H U A X R C
```

Mistletoe

New Years Eve

Carolers

Poinsettia

Zircon

Midwinter

Wreath

Kwanzaa

Swahili

Rose

December Terms 2 - Wordsearch

P	C	X	T	O	X	Q	J	Q	F	Z	W	R	O	Q	R	Z	P
H	Z	R	J	J	O	T	W	D	Z	B	Z	U	G	I	U	R	C
W	S	P	D	O	P	B	W	P	C	L	T	K	I	C	G	W	H
O	J	Z	F	P	C	W	K	N	D	O	H	D	N	H	W	I	K
A	V	D	M	Y	A	A	E	M	K	J	F	B	G	A	L	C	S
J	B	E	Z	T	B	S	B	Y	S	D	Y	X	E	M	U	B	S
P	X	L	F	F	M	S	M	B	M	I	I	T	R	P	W	U	D
W	H	A	V	N	H	A	E	M	F	F	Q	C	B	A	X	B	V
U	O	W	B	L	V	I	E	A	P	B	V	L	R	G	C	B	O
R	L	A	P	P	I	L	M	I	L	K	N	V	E	N	Q	L	C
W	L	R	F	Y	L	I	N	L	W	K	X	X	A	E	K	E	I
E	Y	E	W	T	Y	Y	O	M	P	F	G	M	D	O	Y	L	L
I	O	T	Z	B	B	W	B	A	B	E	M	Q	E	D	B	I	L
G	D	M	B	L	B	M	E	N	U	Z	B	S	C	D	K	G	D
H	I	W	Z	P	N	T	L	H	Q	J	I	I	Q	J	M	H	O
T	M	C	C	A	N	D	Y	C	A	N	E	O	L	E	M	T	R
L	X	M	H	T	J	N	E	L	Z	K	R	M	N	L	E	S	W
Q	A	A	P	R	B	Q	F	I	D	R	A	D	P	A	A	W	H

- Champagne
- Delaware
- Bubble Lights
- Holly
- Weight
- Nobel
- Candy Cane
- Mailman
- Gingerbread
- Wassail

December Terms 3 - Wordsearch

R V V Q U E K O T I Z F Y A V K W V
Q Z B E I L X Y P K W Q U Z L O A R
S O U T P R D R E I D E L A R V L I
Z W M D G D R V J H F B I B H L T R
I J G V Q E A V A B G O E G I L V Q
C J S O E D E C E M Y A Y R H C W Q
W C H U M P H R E Y B O G A R T O O
E Q W P Q W A X N Y K Z Y L T C R U
J H A O K W I S A N T A C L A U S M
L Y K P A I D I B C P R W O B O L X
A O L O A N H R Q O W U Y S A I P I
P U K T I D C G Z L X E C M S W Q Y
H Q J A A S H Z K N X I H U D D B U
G J Y T X O C U J R V A N U Q J J V
L P M O U R H O G M X I N G O T P Q
I T R E G Y U L E L O G M J D K U H
E V A S Z G I V B O G M U Y A A O Q
B U Y F E C O W I N T E R X R S Y U

Winter

Santa Claus

Humphrey Bogart

Boxing Day

Windsor

Ivy

Potatoes

Decem

Yule Log

Dreidel

December Terms 4 - Wordsearch

M	V	L	H	C	N	I	N	C	K	E	F	H	E	M	A	U	G	W	N
V	P	V	P	Q	H	K	K	L	B	P	R	E	H	O	E	S	S	Y	A
F	E	K	Z	V	V	A	Z	X	Y	D	D	G	D	F	C	X	C	P	R
S	A	Q	D	V	H	Z	N	X	R	K	N	K	T	I	J	Z	Z	K	C
K	O	F	E	T	Z	Z	G	U	F	S	W	T	K	U	O	U	J	Y	I
I	Y	H	T	J	J	Z	G	U	K	D	T	O	B	Z	L	G	Y	Y	S
E	N	D	Q	W	U	A	L	X	K	A	O	S	U	U	C	I	C	Q	S
N	K	B	H	I	A	I	I	S	O	G	H	I	T	K	T	P	P	K	U
B	K	P	Z	D	G	T	L	K	A	T	S	A	J	E	Q	Q	Y	B	S
R	V	E	J	D	Q	E	C	B	T	G	S	N	A	J	P	I	O	E	Q
S	S	A	K	G	Y	J	X	H	H	M	I	U	O	X	K	H	V	V	K
I	D	R	U	X	H	R	B	B	N	O	G	T	N	W	T	S	E	C	U
V	V	L	W	Q	N	Z	M	C	X	I	O	Y	T	U	F	I	K	N	Q
G	E	H	H	H	C	O	L	D	S	Z	G	A	O	A	V	L	G	B	C
D	Z	A	R	O	H	S	R	N	F	F	M	H	C	A	R	F	A	S	Y
C	U	R	T	C	B	G	L	N	I	R	O	C	T	T	R	I	Y	K	K
V	O	B	Z	C	A	S	M	J	R	P	S	T	K	L	J	V	U	G	E
U	I	O	V	X	T	F	F	A	T	H	E	R	T	I	M	E	V	S	G
P	G	R	V	M	Y	S	I	I	W	W	E	S	M	O	A	R	K	O	S
C	N	U	Z	G	T	M	N	O	B	E	L	P	J	B	I	Z	X	Z	V

Nobel

Sagittarius

Snowflake

Pearl Harbor

Cold

Chanukah

Father Time

St Stephen

Watch Night

Narcissus

Holiday: Christmas Terms 1 - Wordsearch

B	A	L	W	H	C	G	G	S	J	T	N	D	C	X	O	Q
E	Z	L	U	Y	I	U	X	H	W	W	E	E	R	Z	C	C
T	S	C	P	J	Q	M	B	E	D	V	Q	C	F	E	S	H
H	F	X	L	F	E	A	R	P	D	J	S	E	H	C	R	R
L	G	X	J	L	R	N	P	H	Y	U	A	M	P	V	C	I
E	Z	L	W	U	D	G	G	E	G	O	N	B	P	Z	R	S
H	J	K	C	I	Z	E	A	R	V	K	T	E	E	A	C	T
E	V	E	W	E	S	R	R	D	Y	C	A	R	I	Q	G	M
M	Y	Y	L	W	D	E	C	S	P	A	C	Q	A	B	F	A
C	H	H	L	L	C	I	M	H	Y	H	L	S	M	Y	X	S
Z	Z	W	I	F	Y	J	Y	E	V	O	A	J	I	L	E	E
E	P	Q	I	X	T	U	J	G	N	B	U	L	I	U	X	V
V	Q	B	V	Q	E	T	N	E	C	Z	S	E	O	B	O	E
Z	W	V	D	F	J	Q	F	O	S	R	V	L	V	W	X	G
N	I	F	I	S	M	J	J	Q	D	U	N	V	L	E	I	F
I	S	U	H	U	A	S	R	X	Z	B	S	E	T	N	G	R
Q	D	W	Y	T	Z	R	O	Y	W	T	H	S	U	R	M	M

Jelly

Santa Claus

December

Elves

Wise Men

Bethlehem

Shepherds

Manger

Jesus

Christmas Eve

Holiday: Christmas Terms 2 - Wordsearch

T	J	H	Q	L	I	P	F	I	B	E	F	Q	A	O	L	S	H	T	L
N	B	D	V	Z	V	C	B	D	Z	K	L	M	W	I	U	Z	P	W	A
E	X	O	K	P	U	R	O	G	F	F	U	V	T	D	E	O	Y	E	N
T	T	R	G	A	C	H	R	I	S	T	M	A	S	C	A	R	O	L	G
P	O	B	S	A	S	L	E	I	G	H	U	O	O	L	G	V	D	V	E
W	B	O	B	G	U	N	C	Q	W	V	V	R	U	U	G	S	B	E	L
H	H	J	S	J	U	J	V	T	D	Q	H	B	P	Y	P	K	S	O	S
I	U	G	T	Y	F	R	A	N	K	I	N	C	E	N	S	E	R	T	N
T	M	F	W	C	M	S	C	R	O	O	G	E	K	P	L	G	H	F	M
E	U	A	K	R	G	X	Y	K	Z	G	M	D	R	L	P	Z	V	O	Z
C	X	G	A	E	C	F	R	K	H	N	J	I	M	Y	Q	U	E	U	V
H	R	M	N	K	Y	E	U	S	X	Y	P	I	W	H	Y	F	H	J	G
R	C	D	A	H	G	W	D	U	B	B	P	G	O	I	Y	J	J	W	P
I	C	I	H	Y	E	Q	O	J	L	S	I	R	E	D	T	D	V	Y	Q
S	G	R	R	M	J	S	L	C	U	J	Q	I	J	O	C	Y	V	P	A
T	L	R	I	A	G	O	P	J	J	S	Q	N	I	G	Z	O	P	H	I
M	Q	Q	D	X	H	P	H	W	S	V	V	C	B	V	B	P	S	W	K
A	C	S	R	N	M	R	J	J	G	P	O	H	B	N	G	Y	V	S	D
S	N	A	Y	R	H	G	O	L	D	R	I	N	G	S	B	N	G	V	P
N	Y	Z	E	F	B	V	J	K	U	C	I	G	O	Q	J	E	M	K	R

A Christmas Carol

Grinch

Twelve

Sleigh

Gold Rings

Rudolph

Angels

Scrooge

Frankincense

White Christmas

Holiday: Christmas Terms 3 - Wordsearch

```
A Y N O R T H P O L E O C H E Z E M
I J V M X G Q Y Y M I H H U T C D F
C F E F H P R E S E N T R Z O H M R
P G G D O J Q S N J Q H I R B I L O
W C Y D P X Q Q W A W A S T F A W S
V Q M X X O Q J Z R M T T J N X O T
I W O W N B D I H U F M M X E E N Y
E C M L H G M C Z Y G U A C K V D W
L E M G B M E I H K H F S T N T E Y
L U Y S N O U G S I C B T P Z L R D
S X S P G O X M F T M L R T M C F M
T R Y J G O T I E Q L N E J W K U Z
O I F E F T C J N F N E E R Y K L J
C G U R S M X S C G H L T Y J X R K
K E C I C Y V O P J D D L O G L G N
I O H J V S L F U B M A O H E W R B
N Z K R I N U E V I X G Y Q I S W H
G O F C V R W V Q Y L M B E E B X Z
```

Stocking

Mommy

Present

Boxing Day

Chimney

Frosty

Christmas Tree

Mistletoe

North Pole

Wonderful

Holiday: Christmas Terms 4 - Wordsearch

S	J	J	P	U	D	B	G	B	Q	L	V	M	B	E	M	V
I	I	P	O	C	G	Q	R	B	Y	R	R	U	L	L	H	N
R	Z	L	L	L	V	I	J	X	E	G	O	V	I	C	G	U
L	W	C	E	B	L	H	O	E	C	O	C	H	T	A	W	C
M	Q	A	U	N	G	Y	K	S	X	S	M	M	Z	R	K	E
B	S	N	A	E	T	S	F	D	X	M	Y	U	E	O	T	R
E	T	D	B	C	F	N	R	D	A	Q	Z	A	N	L	R	Z
L	N	L	C	P	X	N	I	D	F	D	X	E	K	S	N	R
L	I	E	T	Y	M	W	R	G	H	T	V	O	V	G	Q	C
S	C	S	N	L	B	N	V	R	H	X	Y	E	F	K	F	M
E	H	K	Y	L	E	R	I	W	F	T	Q	R	N	D	O	O
X	O	V	M	K	Y	O	R	R	K	N	Z	N	J	T	T	N
S	L	U	F	P	O	Q	G	F	J	I	M	N	D	W	R	A
K	A	A	D	C	S	X	I	M	I	R	A	C	L	E	E	F
T	S	L	H	G	R	S	N	R	V	Z	I	O	X	Q	N	I
L	O	T	X	A	N	K	I	M	U	D	S	O	T	D	W	X
N	Q	S	P	J	Y	I	A	C	D	O	J	I	N	A	Y	I

Blitzen

Advent

Jolly

Carols

Bells

Silent Night

Virginia

Candles

St Nicholas

Miracle

December Terms 1 - Wordsearch

```
G Y R P B C I R Z Y U V S D Z A X
R O S E H Z W U M K W A N Z A A R
R S X C X N E W Y E A R S E V E Q
R O M D T D Y F H A S W A H I L I
R E I P G H Y Y E K A T W N T Q G
P I S Y F P I M A I F E I S H J F
T O T S M V S B E I K Z N T N G C
X I L I Z M L D S F K B I V D E D
G T E C T I O U J Z X M K R P D J
F C T A O C H F U V W M I M C T N
K N O R I C Y E P M U C B H Y O P
O Z E O J G U H G V F H N U A N N
C Y V L P O I N S E T T I A T S W
Z U J E Z D O X M I D W I N T E R
H B U R F P G W P J A C R H K K S
Q Q G S D W R E A T H J R D S J P
L I L Y Y A F P A Q D H U A X R C
```

Mistletoe

New Years Eve

Carolers

Poinsettia

Zircon

Midwinter

Wreath

Kwanzaa

Swahili

Rose

December Terms 2 - Wordsearch

P C X T O X Q J Q F Z W R O Q R Z P
H Z R J J O T W D Z B Z U G I U R C
W S P D O P B W P C L T K I C G W H
O J Z F P C W K N D O H D N H W I K
A V D M Y A A E M K J F B G A L C S
J B E Z T B S B Y S D Y X E M U B S
P X L F F M S M B M I I T R P W U D
W H A V N H A E M F F Q C B A X B V
U O W B L V I E A P B V L R G C B O
R L A P P I L M I L K N V E N Q L C
W L R F Y L I N L W K X X A E K E I
E Y E W T Y Y O M P F G M D O Y L L
I O T Z B B W B A B E M Q E D B I L
G D M B L B M E N U Z B S C D K G D
H I W Z P N T L H Q J I I Q J M H O
T M C C A N D Y C A N E O L E M T R
L X M H T J N E L Z K R M N L E S W
Q A A P R B Q F I D R A D P A A W H

Champagne
Delaware
Bubble Lights
Holly
Weight
Nobel
Candy Cane
Mailman
Gingerbread
Wassail

December Terms 3 - Wordsearch

R	V	V	Q	U	E	K	O	T	I	Z	F	Y	A	V	K	W	V
Q	Z	B	E	I	L	X	Y	P	K	W	Q	U	Z	L	O	A	R
S	O	U	T	P	R	D	R	E	I	D	E	L	A	R	V	L	I
Z	W	M	D	G	D	R	V	J	H	F	B	I	B	H	L	T	R
I	J	G	V	Q	E	A	V	A	B	G	O	E	G	I	L	V	Q
C	J	S	O	E	D	E	C	E	M	Y	A	Y	R	H	C	W	Q
W	C	H	U	M	P	H	R	E	Y	B	O	G	A	R	T	O	O
E	Q	W	P	Q	W	A	X	N	Y	K	Z	Y	L	T	C	R	U
J	H	A	O	K	W	I	S	A	N	T	A	C	L	A	U	S	M
L	Y	K	P	A	I	D	I	B	C	P	R	W	O	B	O	L	X
A	O	L	O	A	N	H	R	Q	O	W	U	Y	S	A	I	P	I
P	U	K	T	I	D	C	G	Z	L	X	E	C	M	S	W	Q	Y
H	Q	J	A	A	S	H	Z	K	N	X	I	H	U	D	D	B	U
G	J	Y	T	X	O	C	U	J	R	V	A	N	U	Q	J	J	V
L	P	M	O	U	R	H	O	G	M	X	I	N	G	O	T	P	Q
I	T	R	E	G	Y	U	L	E	L	O	G	M	J	D	K	U	H
E	V	A	S	Z	G	I	V	B	O	G	M	U	Y	A	A	O	Q
B	U	Y	F	E	C	O	W	I	N	T	E	R	X	R	S	Y	U

Winter

Santa Claus

Humphrey Bogart

Boxing Day

Windsor

Ivy

Potatoes

Decem

Yule Log

Dreidel

December Terms 4 - Wordsearch

M V L H C N I N C K E F H E M A U G W N
V P V P Q H K K L B P R E H O E S S Y A
F E K Z V V A Z X Y D D G D F C X C P R
S A Q D V H Z N X R K N K T I J Z Z K C
K O F E T Z Z G U F S W T K U O U J Y I
I Y H T J J Z G U K D T O B Z L G Y Y S
E N D Q W U A L X K A O S U U C I C Q S
N K B H I A I I S O G H I T K T P P K U
B K P Z D G T L K A T S A J E Q Q Y B S
R V E J D Q E C B T G S N A J P I O E Q
S S A K G Y J X H H M I U O X K H V V K
I D R U X H R B B N O G T N W T S E C U
V V L W Q N Z M C X I O Y T U F I K N Q
G E H H H C O L D S Z G A O A V L G B C
D Z A R O H S R N F F M H C A R F A S Y
C U R T C B G L N I R O C T T R I Y K K
V O B Z C A S M J R P S T K L J V U G E
U I O V X T F F A T H E R T I M E V S G
P G R V M Y S I I W W E S M O A R K O S
C N U Z G T M N O B E L P J B I Z X Z V

Nobel

Sagittarius

Snowflake

Pearl Harbor

Cold

Chanukah

Father Time

St Stephen

Watch Night

Narcissus

Holiday: Christmas Terms 1 - Wordsearch

B	A	L	W	H	C	G	G	S	J	T	N	D	C	X	O	Q
E	Z	L	U	Y	I	U	X	H	W	W	E	E	R	Z	C	C
T	S	C	P	J	Q	M	B	E	D	V	Q	C	F	E	S	H
H	F	X	L	F	E	A	R	P	D	J	S	E	H	C	R	R
L	G	X	J	L	R	N	P	H	Y	U	A	M	P	V	C	I
E	Z	L	W	U	D	G	G	E	G	O	N	B	P	Z	R	S
H	J	K	C	I	Z	E	A	R	V	K	T	E	E	A	C	T
E	V	E	W	E	S	R	R	D	Y	C	A	R	I	Q	G	M
M	Y	Y	L	W	D	E	C	S	P	A	C	Q	A	B	F	A
C	H	H	L	L	C	I	M	H	Y	H	L	S	M	Y	X	S
Z	Z	W	I	F	Y	J	Y	E	V	O	A	J	I	L	E	E
E	P	Q	I	X	T	U	J	G	N	B	U	L	I	U	X	V
V	Q	B	V	Q	E	T	N	E	C	Z	S	E	O	B	O	E
Z	W	V	D	F	J	Q	F	O	S	R	V	L	V	W	X	G
N	I	F	I	S	M	J	J	Q	D	U	N	V	L	E	I	F
I	S	U	H	U	A	S	R	X	Z	B	S	E	T	N	G	R
Q	D	W	Y	T	Z	R	O	Y	W	T	H	S	U	R	M	M

Jelly

Santa Claus

December

Elves

Wise Men

Bethlehem

Shepherds

Manger

Jesus

Christmas Eve

Holiday: Christmas Terms 2 - Wordsearch

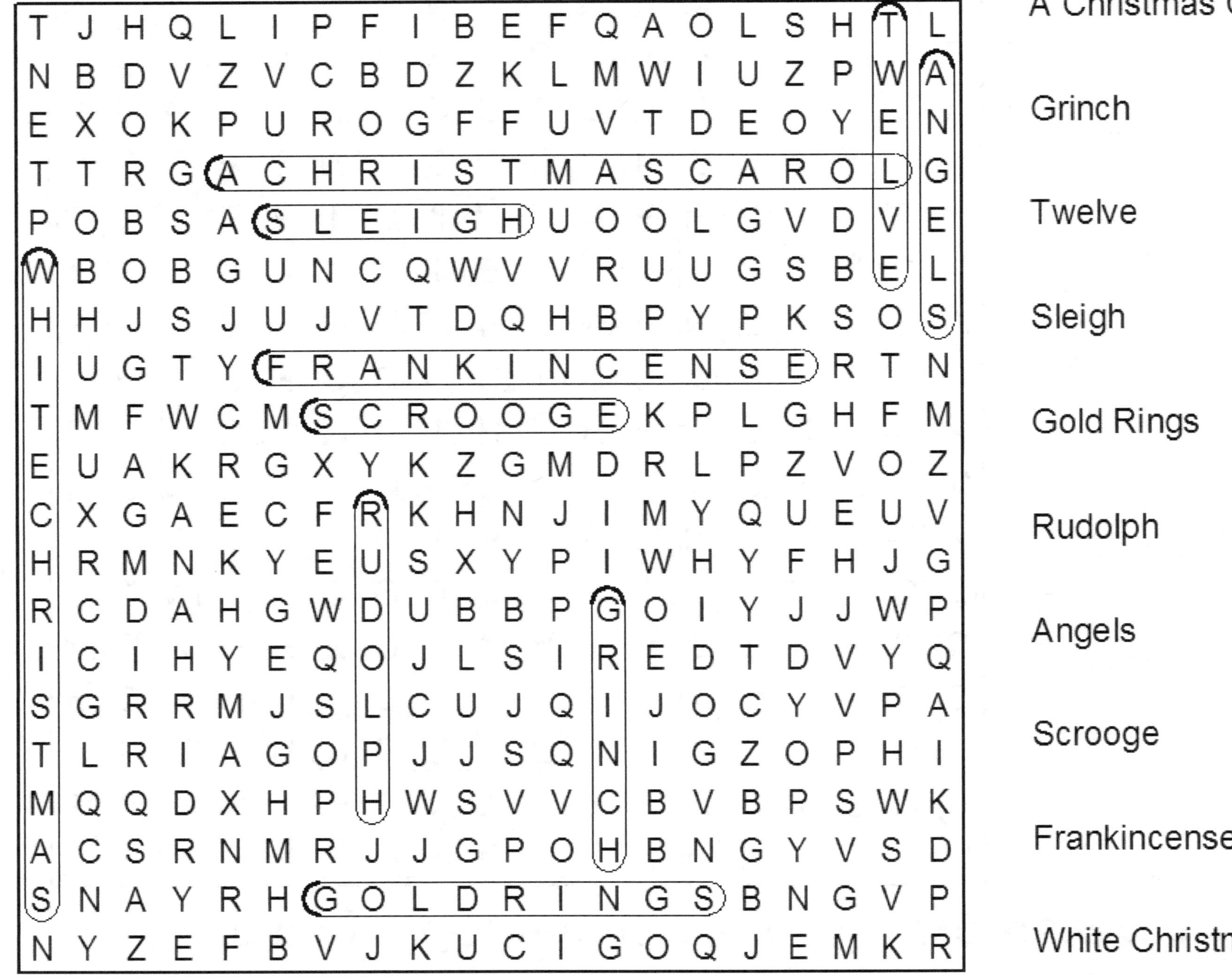

A Christmas Carol

Grinch

Twelve

Sleigh

Gold Rings

Rudolph

Angels

Scrooge

Frankincense

White Christmas

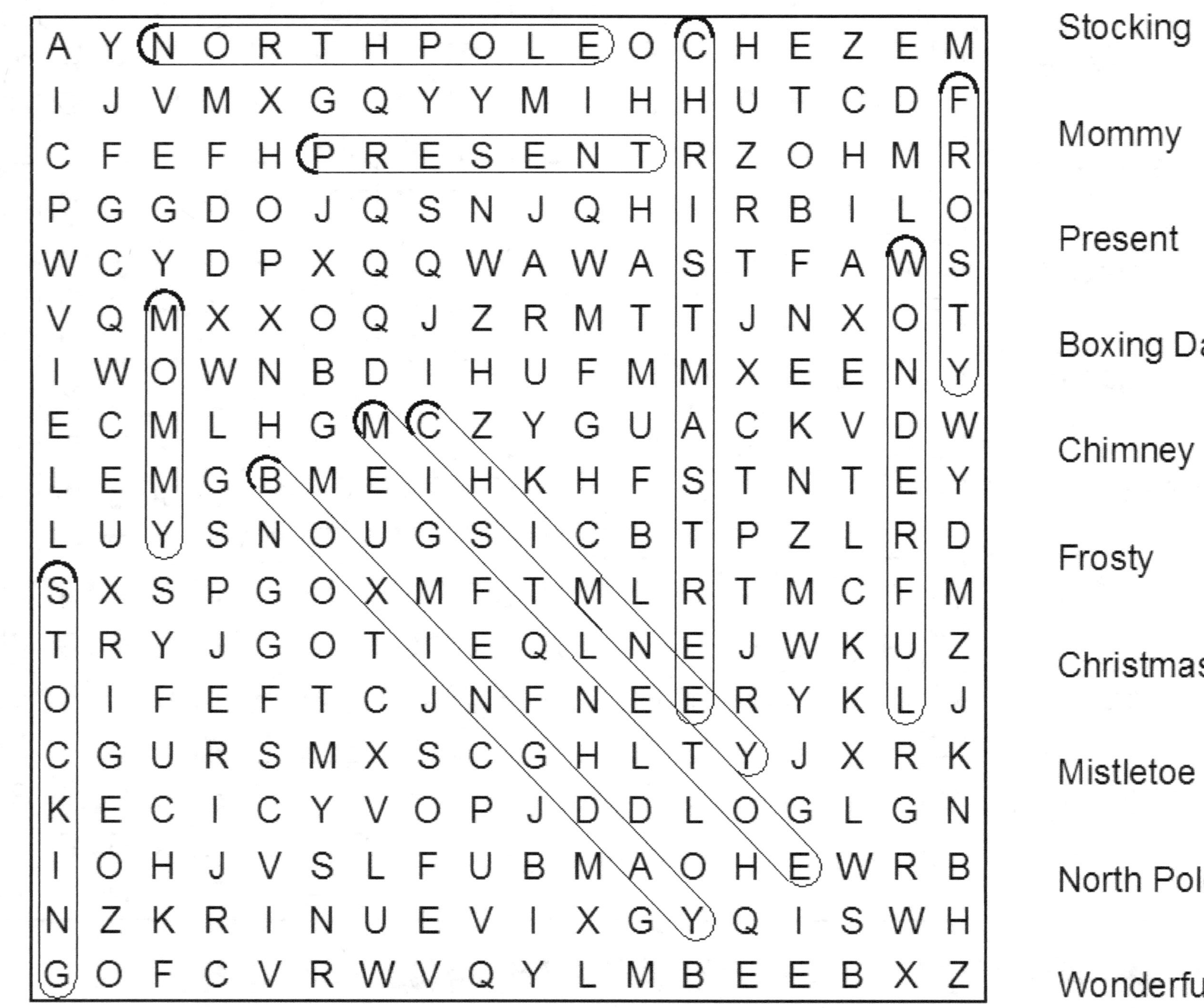
Holiday: Christmas Terms 3 - Wordsearch
A Y N O R T H P O L E O C H E Z E M
I J V M X G Q Y Y M I H H U T C D F
C F E F H P R E S E N T R Z O H M R
P G G D O J Q S N J Q H I R B I L O
W C Y D P X Q Q W A W A S T F A W S
V Q M X X O Q J Z R M T T J N X O T
I W O W N B D I H U F M M X E E N Y
E C M L H G M C Z Y G U A C K V D W
L E M G B M E I H K H F S T N T E Y
L U Y S N O U G S I C B T P Z L R D
S X S P G O X M F T M L R T M C F M
T R Y J G O T I E Q L N E J W K U Z
O I F E F T C J N F N E E R Y K L J
C G U R S M X S C G H L T Y J X R K
K E C I C Y V O P J D D L O G L G N
I O H J V S L F U B M A O H E W R B
N Z K R I N U E V I X G Y Q I S W H
G O F C V R W V Q Y L M B E E B X Z
Stocking
Mommy
Present
Boxing Day
Chimney
Frosty
Christmas Tree
Mistletoe
North Pole
Wonderful

Holiday: Christmas Terms 4 - Wordsearch

```
S J J P U D B G B Q L V M B E M V
I I P O C G Q R B Y R R U L L H N
R Z L L L V I J X E G O V I C G U
L W C E B L H O E C O C H T A W C
M Q A U N G Y K S X S M M Z R K E
B S N A E T S F D X M Y U E O T R
E T D B C F N R D A Q Z A N L R Z
L N L C P X N I D F D X E K S N R
L I E T Y M W R G H T V O V G Q C
S C S N L B N V R H X Y E F K F M
E H K Y L E R I W F T Q R N D O O
X O V M K Y O R R K N Z N J T T N
S L U F P O Q G F J I M N D W R A
K A A D C S X I M I R A C L E E F
T S L H G R S N R V Z I O X Q N I
L O T X A N K I M U D S O T D W X
N Q S P J Y I A C D O J I N A Y I
```

Blitzen

Advent

Jolly

Carols

Bells

Silent Night

Virginia

Candles

St Nicholas

Miracle

Activity Lesson Plans

December and Christmas Crossword

December and Christmas Crossword

- The following pages contain basic templates that can be used by anyone. The leader must allow for the participant to be successful.
- The leader should read all step-by-step directions of an Activity Outline before beginning an activity with a participant. The step-by-step directions are general guidelines for the leader/caregiver to use and potentially modify in order to help the participant successfully engage in the chosen activity.
- The leader must always be present when engaging the participant in an activity.
- The leader must take all necessary and reasonable precautions to ensure the safety of the participant.
- The leader should have necessary materials ready and prepared prior to the beginning of the activity.
- To ensure that the participant reaps the benefits of being engaged, please adapt any and all activities to the participants functional level.

Program Name: December Crossword **Date:** ______________

Leader: ____ **Time:** ______________

Objective:

- Stimulate cognitive functioning
- Increase self-worth and improve self-esteem
- Increase socialization
- Foster friendship, laughter and closeness
- Provide a sense of accomplishment
- Stimulate memory
- Have some fun!

Materials:

- Flat surface for participant to write on
- Templates on the following pages provided
- Pen, pencil or high lighter

Note: If a participant is in a bed, recliner or wheelchair, consider using the R.O.S. Multi-Purpose Board Insert and the R.O.S. Legacy™ System Console available at R.O.S. Therapy Systems (www.therosstore.com) as an option for a flat surface to allow the participant the opportunity to fully engage in this activity.

Prerequisite Skills:

Every person has his or her own unique physical/cognitive abilities and needs. How a participant responds to an activity will dictate how the caregiver will modify or adapt a Lesson Plan to meet individual client needs and abilities – now and in the future.

Program Name: December Crossword **Date:** ____________

Leader: ______________________________ **Time:** ____________

Activity Outline:

The leader explains to the participant that they will be working on a Crossword puzzle.

1. Use the following templates to enjoy a Crossword based on topics of interest.

Option 1: Based on the participants abilities, the participant completes an activity on their own.

Option 2: Based on the participants abilities, the leader assists with finding answers.

Option 3: Based on the participants abilities, the leader and the participant have a discussion based on words and topics included in this activity.

Evaluation:

December Terms 1 - Crossword

Across

5. Language the word "Kwanzaa" is taken from
6. Last night of the year
9. Halfway through the season, it was bleak in the long ago carol
10. Flower rare to find in December, according to the quote

Down

1. Plant shot out of a tree in December
2. You might find them singing outside your door in December
3. Christmas plant with red leaves
4. Week-long celebration of African heritage & traditions
7. Alternative December birthstone
8. It's on the door in December

December Terms 2 - Crossword

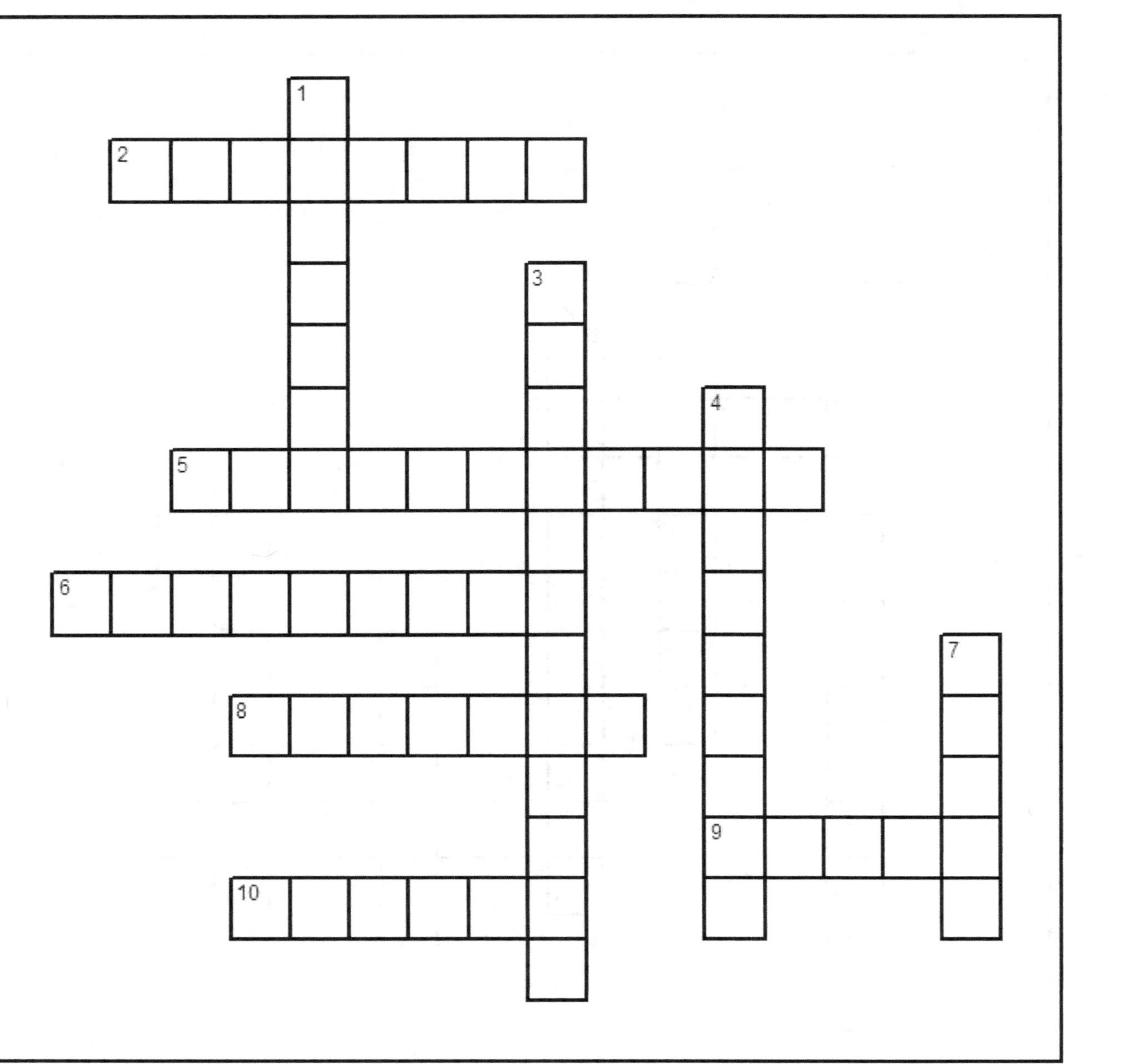

Across

2. The first state
5. Cookie men are made of this
6. Traditional December 31 beverage
8. Traditional English holiday drink
9. His prize is awarded on his December death anniversary
10. What might increase if you eat too many sweets

Down

1. He delivers Christmas cards
3. Christmas lights popular during the 50's and 60's
4. Red and white striped hooked candy
7. Berry-laden December plant

December Terms 3 - Crossword

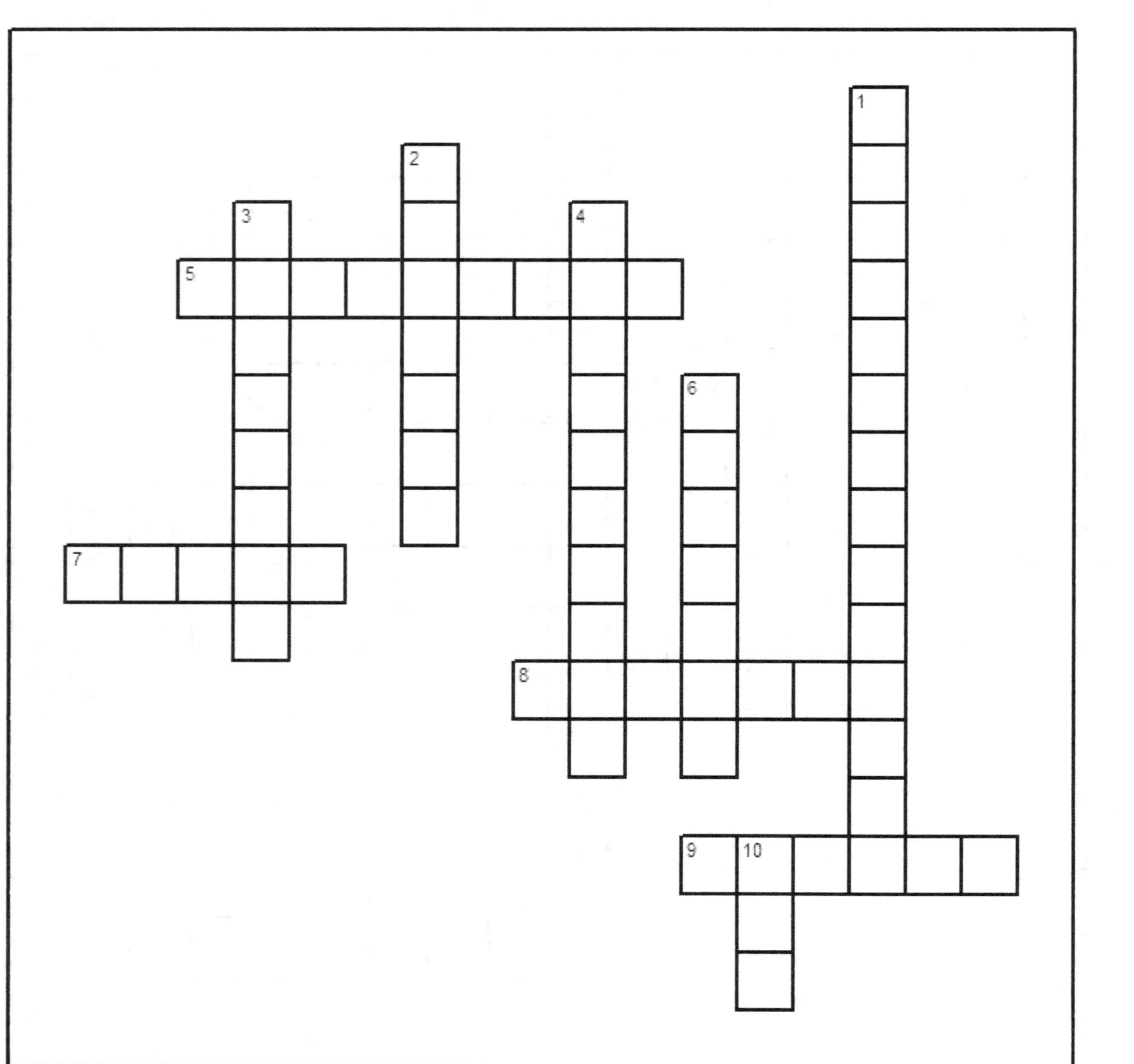

Across

5. Celebration Muhammad Ali might enjoy
7. Latin prefix for "ten"
8. Its embers scare away evil spirits
9. Season begins December 21

Down

1. He might've looked at you, kid, on his Christmas birthday
2. This duke abdicated the English throne in December
3. What latkes are made of
4. He visits December 24
6. Chanukah toy
10. Plant holly is often paired with

December Terms 4 - Crossword

Across

2. Greek god who loved looking at himself
3. How December weather feels
5. He leaves for good on New Year's Eve
7. Worship service held late December 31
8. TNT inventor with a December Birthday
9. His feast day is December 26

Down

1. Might be caught on the tongue in December
3. Alternate spelling for the Festival of Lights
4. Was bombed on December 7, 1941
6. Celestial Hunter, December zodiac

Holiday: Christmas Terms 1 - Crossword

Across

1. Month Christmas is celebrated
4. Watching their flocks when Jesus was born
6. Town where Jesus was born
8. He brings gifts on Christmas Eve
9. Santa's belly shakes like bowl full of _ _ _ _ _
10. They came from a far to see Jesus

Down

2. Mary laid Jesus in one of these
3. The night before Christmas
5. We celebrate His birthday on Christmas
7. Makers of Santa's toys

Holiday: Christmas Terms 2 - Crossword

1 2 3 4 5 6 7 8 9 10

Across

1. Miser in "A Christmas Carol"
4. Santa rides in this
5. A red-nosed reindeer
6. He stole Christmas
7. One of the Wise Men's gifts to Jesus
9. Charles Dickens classic tale about a miser
10. Announced Jesus's birth from the sky

Down

2. Given on the 5th day of Christmas
3. Bing Crosby sang a song about this
8. Number of days celebrated after Christmas

Holiday: Christmas Terms 3 - Crossword

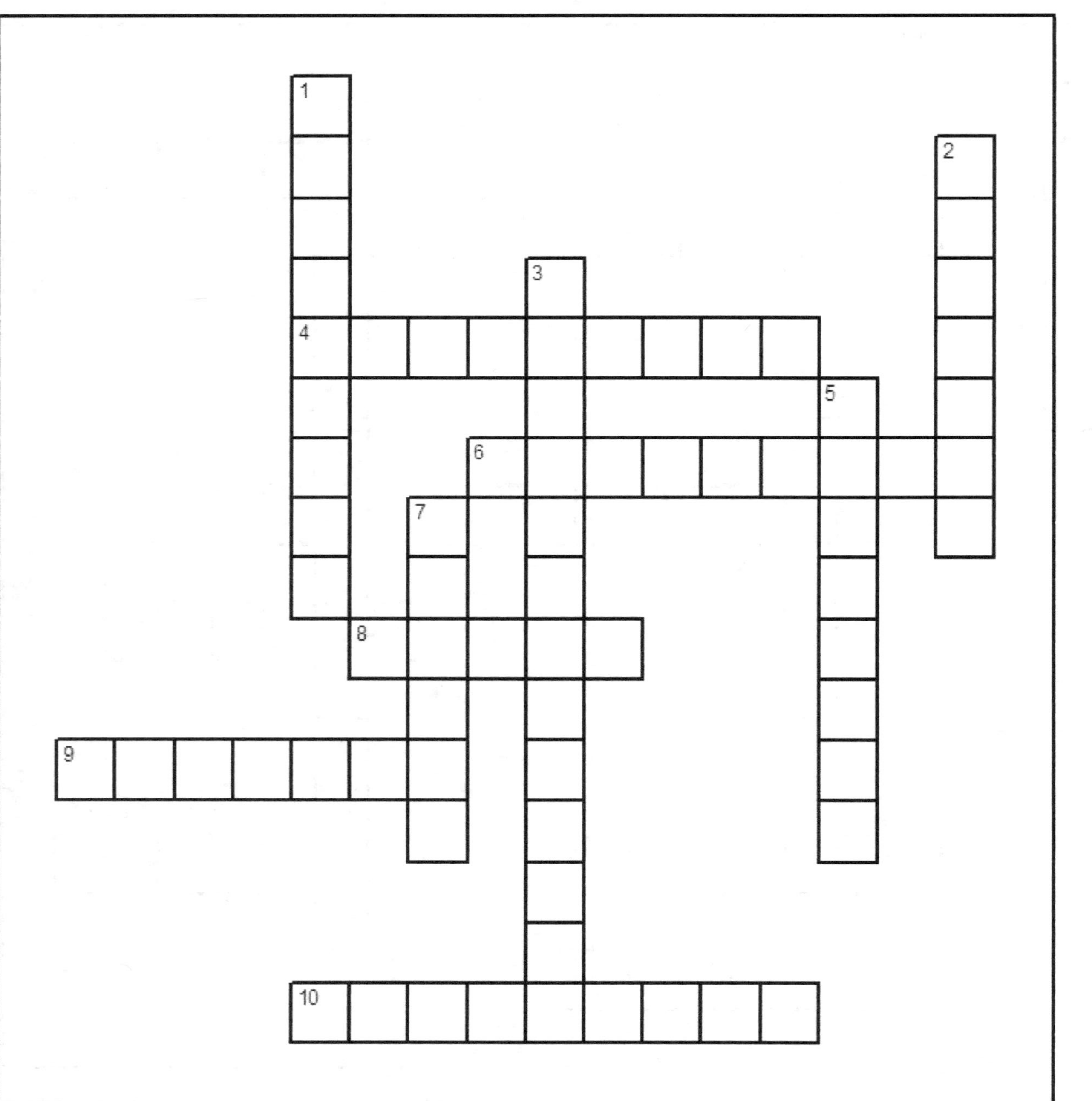

Across

4. Place where Santa lives
6. People kiss under this
8. She kissed Santa Claus
9. Item exchanged at Christmas
10. "It's a __________ Life"

Down

1. Celebrated by the British on December 26
2. Where Santa enters the house
3. Evergreen decorated for the holidays
5. Santa fills this with candy and small items
7. Snowman who wore a magic hat

Holiday: Christmas Terms 4 - Crossword

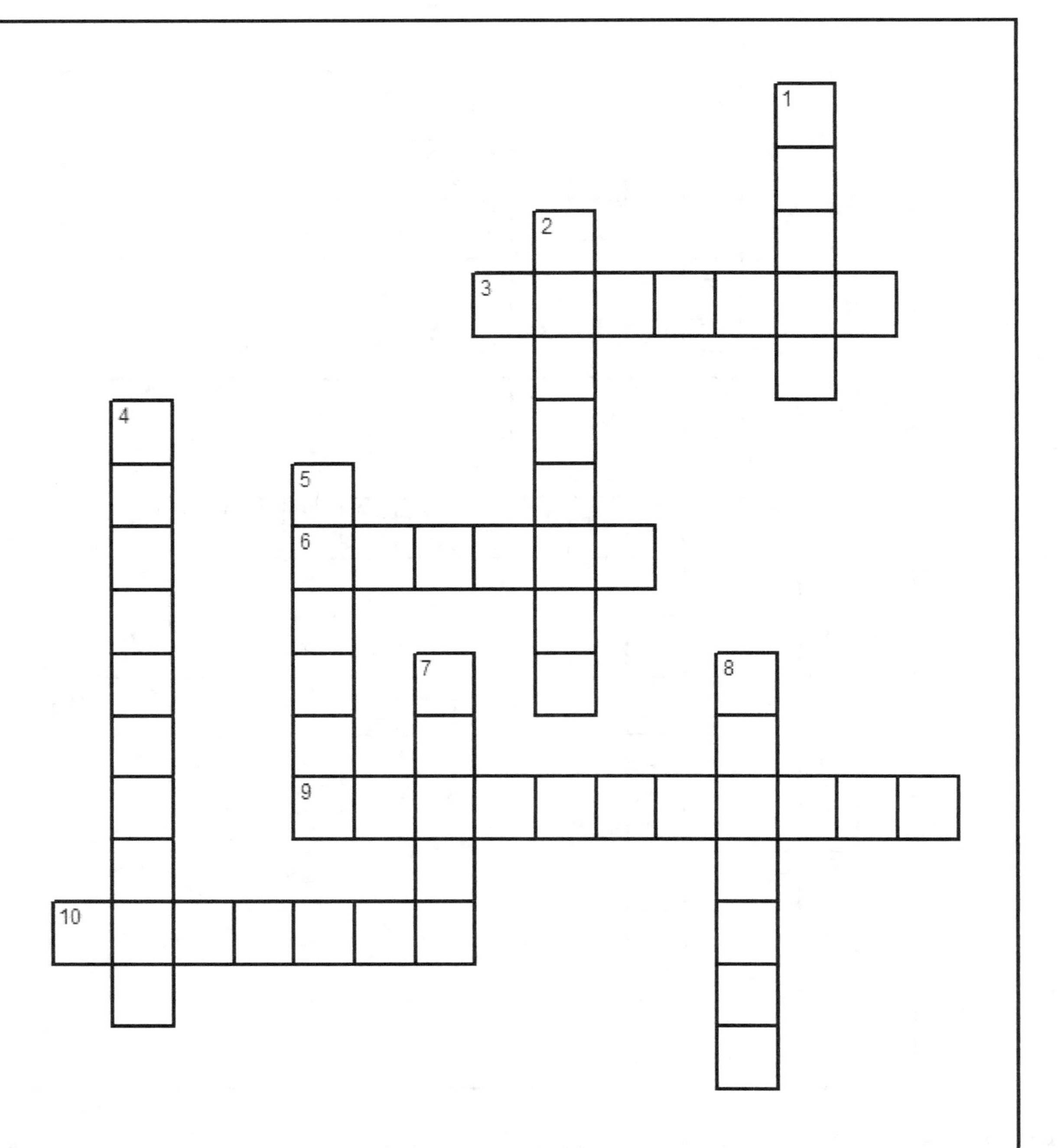

Across

3. This happened on 34th Street
6. Season celebrated before Christmas Day
9. Carol about a very quiet evening
10. A symbol of light

Down

1. St. Nicholas was said to be this
2. She wasn't sure if there was a Santa Claus
4. Another name for Santa Claus
5. Songs about Christmas
7. Instrument rung at Christmas
8. One of Santa's reindeer

December Terms 1 - Crossword

													1 M
										2 C			I
										A			S
				3 P						R			T
	4 K			O						O			L
5 S	W	A	H	I	L	I				L			E
	A			N						E			T
	N			S						R			O
	Z		6 N	E	W	Y	E	A	R	S	E	V	E
	A			T									
	A			T			7 Z				8 W		
			9 M	I	D	W	I	N	T	E	R		
				A			R				E		
							C				A		
						10 R	O	S	E		T		
							N				H		

Across

5. Language the word "Kwanzaa" is taken from
6. Last night of the year
9. Halfway through the season, it was bleak in the long ago carol
10. Flower rare to find in December, according to the quote

Down

1. Plant shot out of a tree in December
2. You might find them singing outside your door in December
3. Christmas plant with red leaves
4. Week-long celebration of African heritage & traditions
7. Alternative December birthstone
8. It's on the door in December

December Terms 2 - Crossword

				M											
	D	E	L	A	W	A	R	E							
				I											
				L				B							
				M				U							
				A				B			C				
		G	I	N	G	E	R	B	R	E	A	D			
								L			N				
C	H	A	M	P	A	G	N	E			D				
								L			Y				H
			W	A	S	S	A	I	L		C				O
								G			A				L
								H			N	O	B	E	L
			W	E	I	G	H	T			E				Y
								S							

Across

2. The first state
5. Cookie men are made of this
6. Traditional December 31 beverage
8. Traditional English holiday drink
9. His prize is awarded on his December death anniversary
10. What might increase if you eat too many sweets

Down

1. He delivers Christmas cards
3. Christmas lights popular during the 50's and 60's
4. Red and white striped hooked candy
7. Berry-laden December plant

December Terms 3 - Crossword

														1 H		
						2 W								U		
			3 P			I			4 S					M		
		5 B	O	X	I	N	G	D	A	Y				P		
			T			D			N					H		
			A			S			T		6 D			R		
			T			O			A		R			E		
			O			R			C		E			Y		
7 D	E	C	E	M					L		I			B		
			S						A		D			O		
								8 Y	U	L	E	L	O	G		
									S		L			A		
														R		
											9 W	10 I	N	T	E	R
												V				
												Y				

Across

5. Celebration Muhammad Ali might enjoy
7. Latin prefix for "ten"
8. Its embers scare away evil spirits
9. Season begins December 21

Down

1. He might've looked at you, kid, on his Christmas birthday
2. This duke abdicated the English throne in December
3. What latkes are made of
4. He visits December 24
6. Chanukah toy
10. Plant holly is often paired with

December Terms 4 - Crossword

```
 S
 NARCISSUS
 O
 W           COLD
 F           H
 L       P   A
FATHERTIME   N
 K       A   U
 E       R   K
      S  L   A
     WATCHNIGHT
      G  A
      I  R
      T  B
      T NOBEL
      A  R
      R
      I
      U
      STSTEPHEN
```

Across

2. Greek god who loved looking at himself
3. How December weather feels
5. He leaves for good on New Year's Eve
7. Worship service held late December 31
8. TNT inventor with a December Birthday
9. His feast day is December 26

Down

1. Might be caught on the tongue in December
3. Alternate spelling for the Festival of Lights
4. Was bombed on December 7, 1941
6. Celestial Hunter, December zodiac

Holiday: Christmas Terms 1 - Crossword

```
     DECEMBER
         A
         N
     C   G
    SHEPHERDS
     R   R
     I
     S        J
   BETHLEHEM  E
     M        S
     A     E  U
     SANTACLAUS
     E     V
     V    JELLY
WISEMEN    S
```

Across

1. Month Christmas is celebrated
4. Watching their flocks when Jesus was born
6. Town where Jesus was born
8. He brings gifts on Christmas Eve
9. Santa's belly shakes like bowl full of _ _ _ _ _
10. They came from a far to see Jesus

Down

2. Mary laid Jesus in one of these
3. The night before Christmas
5. We celebrate His birthday on Christmas
7. Makers of Santa's toys

Holiday: Christmas Terms 2 - Crossword

									1 S	C	R	O	O	2 G	E				
					3 W									O					
4 S	L	E	I	G	H					5 R	U	D	O	L	P	H			
					I									D					
					T									R					
					E									I					
	6 G	R	I	N	C	H								N					
					H									G					
				7 F	R	A	N	K	I	N	C	E	N	S	E				
					I														
					S														8 T
					T														W
					M														E
					9 A	C	H	R	I	S	T	M	A	S	C	A	R	O	L
10 A	N	G	E	L	S														V
																			E

Across

1. Miser in "A Christmas Carol"
4. Santa rides in this
5. A red-nosed reindeer
6. He stole Christmas
7. One of the Wise Men's gifts to Jesus
9. Charles Dickens classic tale about a miser
10. Announced Jesus's birth from the sky

Down

2. Given on the 5th day of Christmas
3. Bing Crosby sang a song about this
8. Number of days celebrated after Christmas

Holiday: Christmas Terms 3 - Crossword

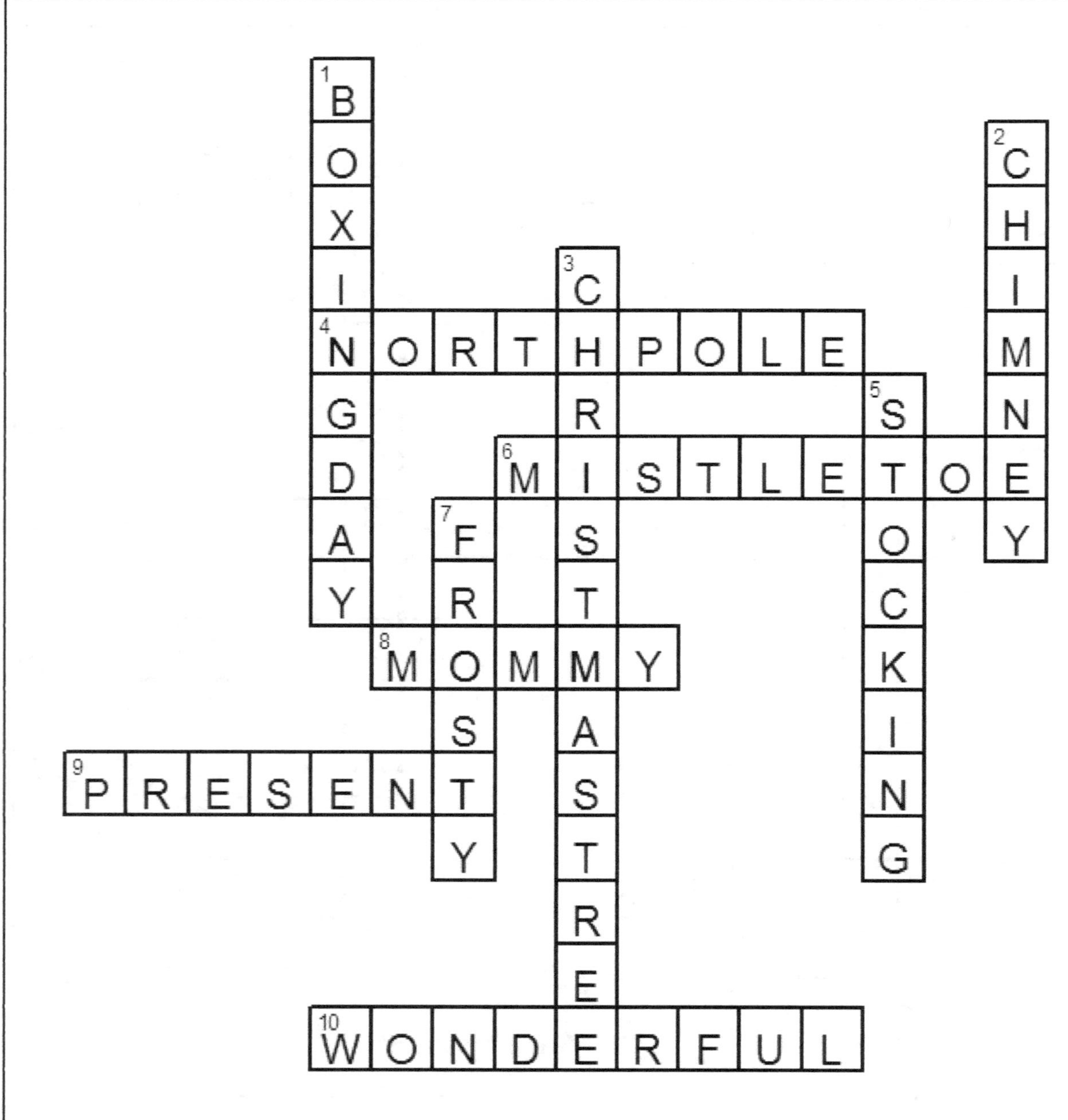

Across

4. Place where Santa lives
6. People kiss under this
8. She kissed Santa Claus
9. Item exchanged at Christmas
10. "It's a __________ Life"

Down

1. Celebrated by the British on December 26
2. Where Santa enters the house
3. Evergreen decorated for the holidays
5. Santa fills this with candy and small items
7. Snowman who wore a magic hat

Holiday: Christmas Terms 4 - Crossword

												1 J		
												O		
								2 V				L		
							3 M	I	R	A	C	L	E	
								R				Y		
	4 S							G						
	T			5 C				I						
	N			6 A	D	V	E	N	T					
	I			R				I						
	C			O		7 B		A			8 B			
	H			L		E					L			
	O			9 S	I	L	E	N	T	N	I	G	H	T
	L					L					T			
10 C	A	N	D	L	E	S					Z			
	S										E			
											N			

Across

3. This happened on 34th Street
6. Season celebrated before Christmas Day
9. Carol about a very quiet evening
10. A symbol of light

Down

1. St. Nicholas was said to be this
2. She wasn't sure if there was a Santa Claus
4. Another name for Santa Claus
5. Songs about Christmas
7. Instrument rung at Christmas
8. One of Santa's reindeer

Activity Lesson Plans

December and Christmas Code Breakers

December and Christmas Code Breakers

- The following pages contain basic templates that can be used by anyone. The leader must allow for the participant to be successful.
- The leader should read all step-by-step directions of an Activity Outline before beginning an activity with a participant. The step-by-step directions are general guidelines for the leader/ caregiver to use and potentially modify in order to help the participant successfully engage in the chosen activity.
- The leader must always be present when engaging the participant in an activity.
- The leader must take all necessary and reasonable precautions to ensure the safety of the participant.
- The leader should have necessary materials ready and prepared prior to the beginning of the activity.
- To ensure that the participant reaps the benefits of being engaged, please adapt any and all activities to the participants functional level.

Program Name: December Code Breakers **Date:** ____________

Leader: ________________________________ **Time:** ____________

Objective:

- Stimulate cognitive functioning
- Increase self-worth and improve self-esteem
- Increase socialization
- Foster friendship, laughter and closeness
- Provide a sense of accomplishment
- Stimulate memory
- Have some fun!

Materials:

- Flat surface for participant to write on
- Templates on the following pages provided
- Pen, pencil or high lighter

Note: If a participant is in a bed, recliner or wheelchair, consider using the R.O.S. Multi-Purpose Board Insert and the R.O.S. Legacy™ System Console available at R.O.S. Therapy Systems (www.therosstore.com) as an option for a flat surface to allow the participant the opportunity to fully engage in this activity.

Prerequisite Skills:

Every person has his or her own unique physical/cognitive abilities and needs. How a participant responds to an activity will dictate how the caregiver will modify or adapt a Lesson Plan to meet individual client needs and abilities – now and in the future.

Program Name: December Code Breakers **Date:** ____________

Leader: ________________________________ **Time:** ____________

Activity Outline:

The leader explains to the participant that they will be working on Code Breaker puzzles.

1. Use the following templates to enjoy code breaker puzzles based on topics of interest.

Option 1: Based on the participants abilities, the participant completes an activity on their own.

Option 2: Based on the participants abilities, the leader assists with finding answers.

Option 3: Based on the participant abilities, the leader and the participant have a discussion based on words and topics included in this activity.

Evaluation:

CodeBreaker

Use the telephone dial pad and place the correct letter above each number to break the code and solve the

December Mysteries

#1 North America's shortest day of the year

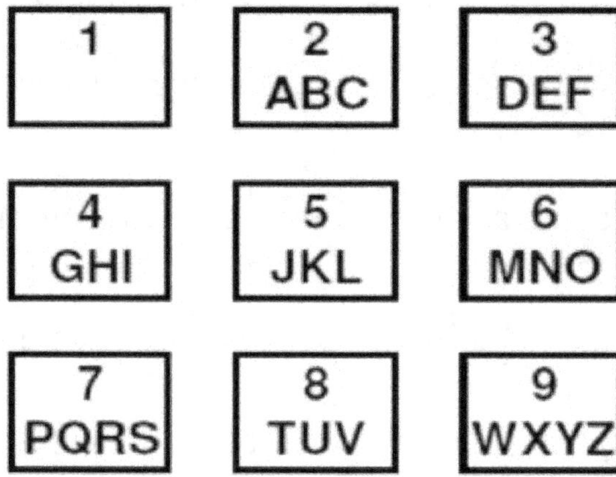

W _ _ _ _ _   _ _ _ _ _ _ _ _

9 4 6 8 3 7   7 6 5 7 8 2 2 3

#2 People kiss under the December plant

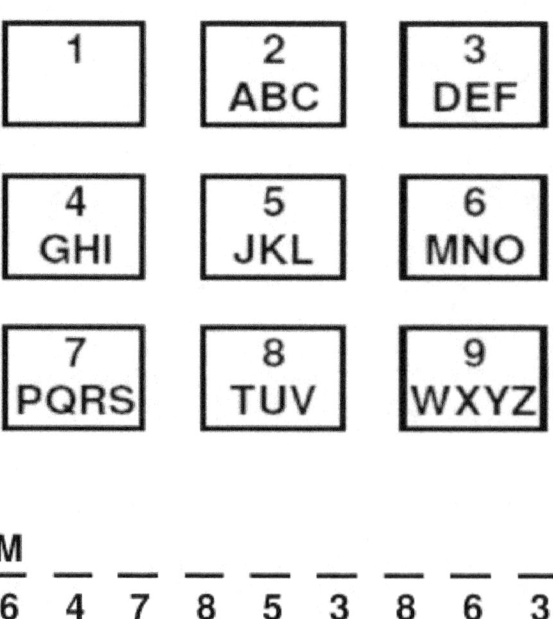

M _ _ _ _ _ _ _ _

6 4 7 8 5 3 8 6 3

CodeBreaker

Use the telephone dial pad and place the correct letter above each number to break the code and solve the

December Mysteries

#3 This good king looked down on the feast of Stephen

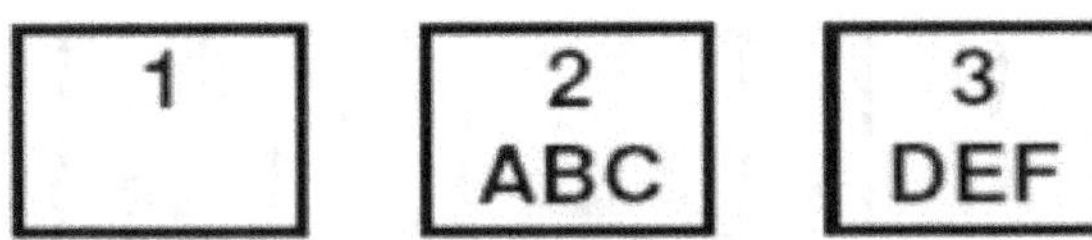

4 GHI | 5 JKL | 6 MNO

7 PQRS | 8 TUV | 9 WXYZ

W _ _ _ _ _ _ _ _

9 3 6 2 3 7 5 2 7

#4 Another name for Hannukkah

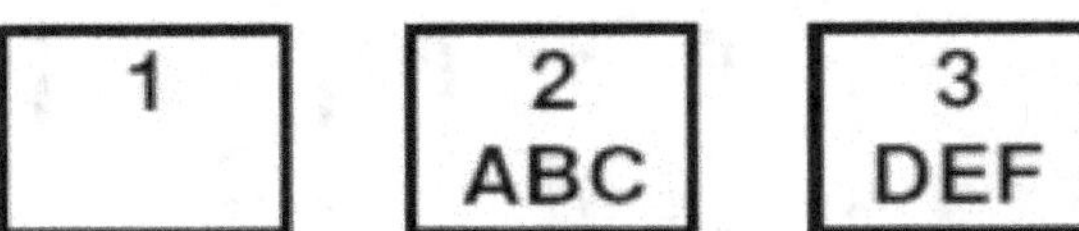

4 GHI | 5 JKL | 6 MNO

7 PQRS | 8 TUV | 9 WXYZ

F _ _ _ _ _ _ _   _ _   _ _ _ _ _ _

3 3 7 8 4 8 2 5   6 3   5 4 4 4 8 7

CodeBreaker

Use the telephone dial pad and place the correct letter above each number to break the code and solve the

December Mysteries

#5 Bombed on a day which will live in infamy

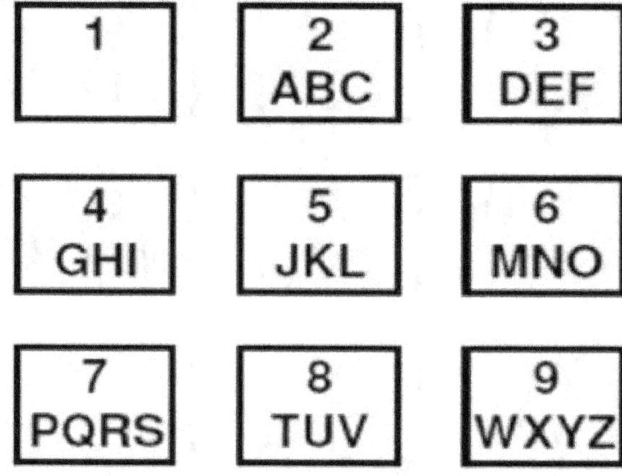

P _ _ _ _   _ _ _ _ _ _

7 3 2 7 5   4 2 7 2 6 7

#6 December is the 12th month in the calendar

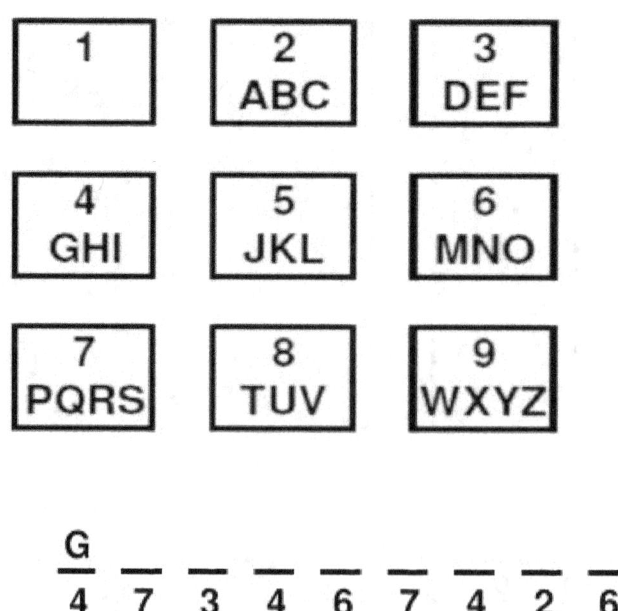

G _ _ _ _ _ _ _ _

4 7 3 4 6 7 4 2 6

CodeBreaker

Use the telephone dial pad and place the correct letter above each number to break the code and solve the

Awesome December Mysteries

#1 He introduced this red leafed plant from Mexico

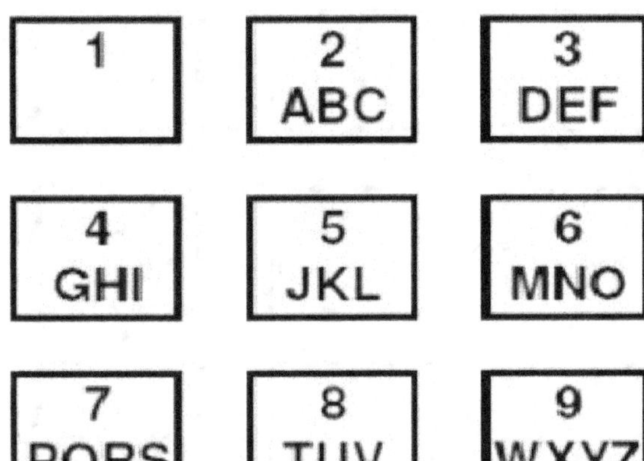

J _ _ _   **P** _ _ _ _ _ _ _

5 6 3 5   7 6 4 6 7 3 8 8

#2 Where you might be at midnight on December 24th

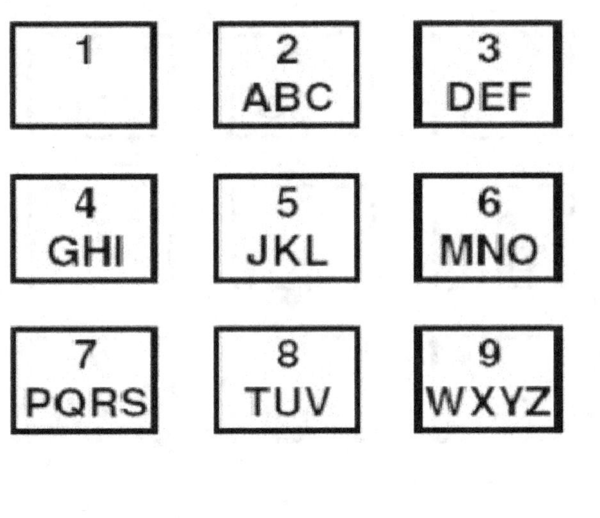

M _ _ _ _ _ _ _   _ _ _ _

6 4 3 6 4 4 4 8   6 2 7 7

CodeBreaker

Use the telephone dial pad and place the correct letter above each number to break the code and solve the

Awesome December Mysteries

#3 Jimmy Stewart and Donna Reed star in this classic movie

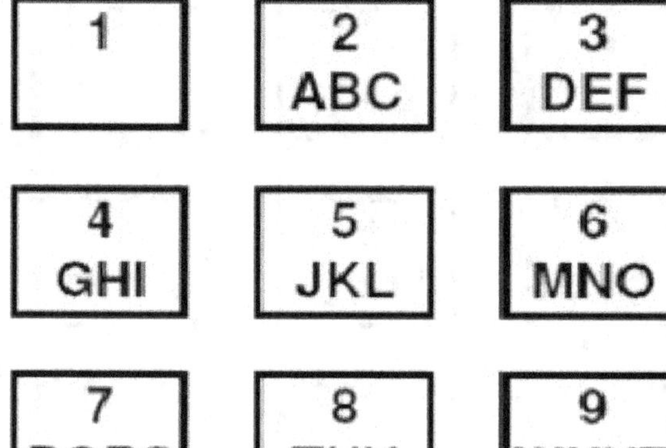

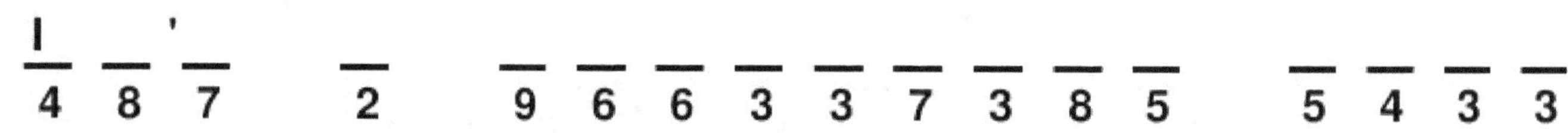

#4 December event that flavored a harbor

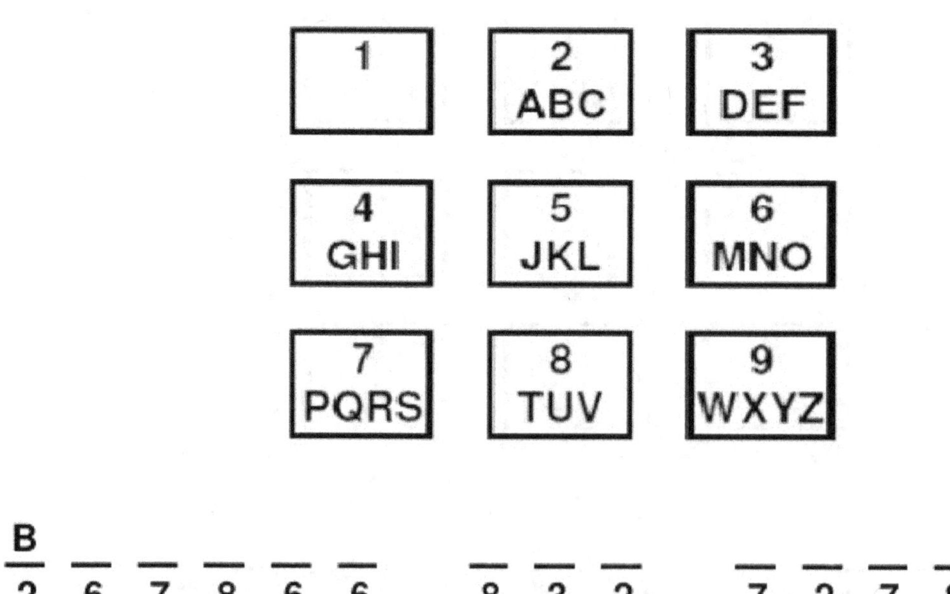

B

2 6 7 8 6 6 8 3 2 7 2 7 8 9

CodeBreaker

Use the telephone dial pad and place the correct letter above each number to break the code and solve the

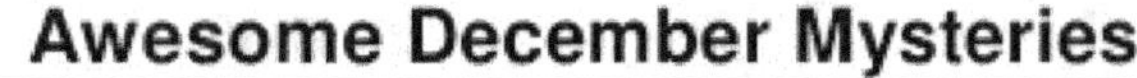

Awesome December Mysteries

#5 Mustachioed comedian who died
25-Dec-77

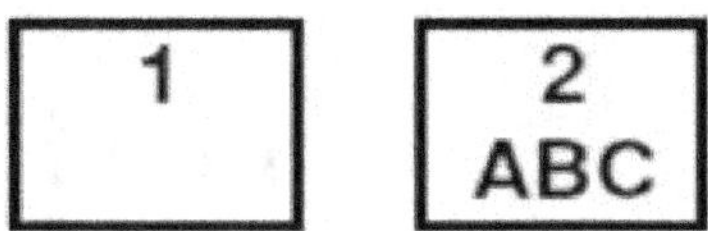

1	2 ABC	3 DEF
4 GHI	5 JKL	6 MNO
7 PQRS	8 TUV	9 WXYZ

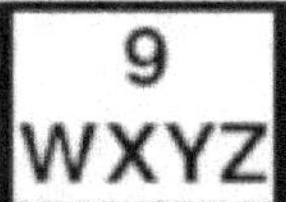

C _ _ _ _ _ _ C _ _ _ _ _ _
2 4 2 7 5 4 3 2 4 2 7 5 4 6

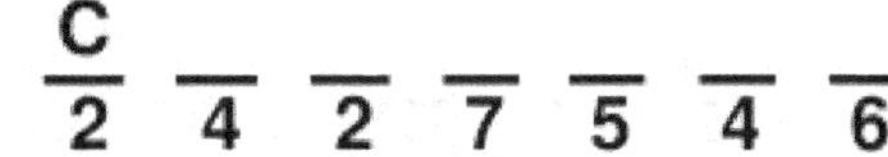

#6 Movie with famous line about a BB Gun
"You'll shoot your eye out"

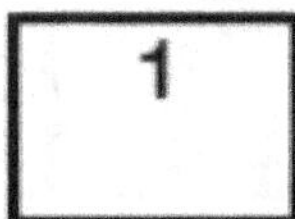

1	2 ABC	3 DEF
4 GHI	5 JKL	6 MNO
7 PQRS	8 TUV	9 WXYZ

A _ _ _ _ _ _ _ _ _ _ _ _ _ _
2 2 4 7 4 7 8 6 2 7 7 8 6 7 9

CodeBreaker

Use the telephone dial pad and place the correct letter above each number to break the code and solve the

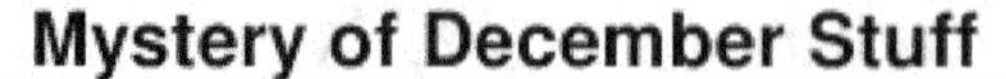

Mystery of December Stuff

#1 Famous blue eyed singer born in December

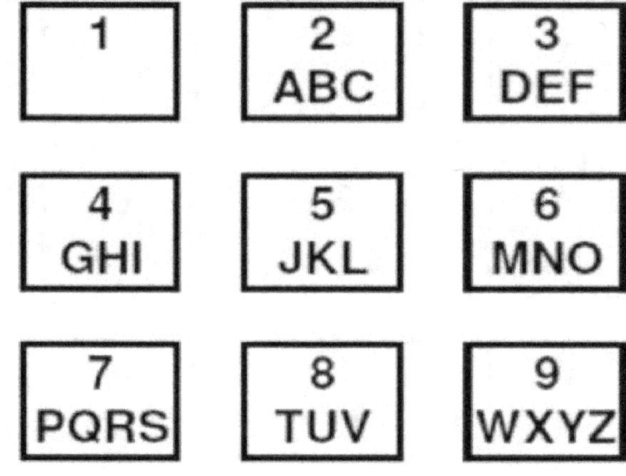

F _ _ _ _   _ _ _ _ _ _ _

3 7 2 6 5   7 4 6 2 8 7 2

#2 They took flight in 1903

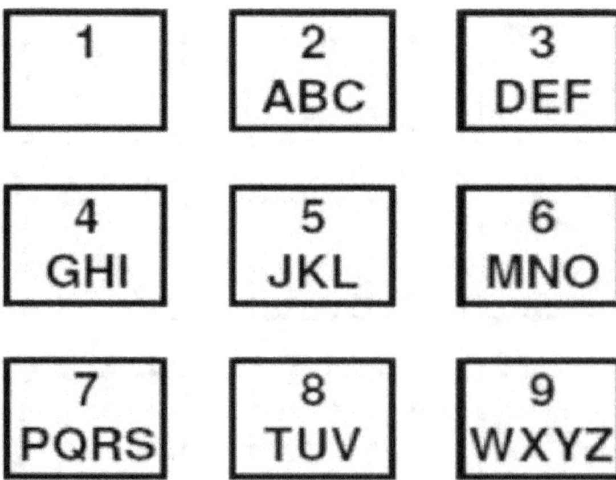

W _ _ _ _ _   _ _ _ _ _ _ _ _

9 7 4 4 4 8   2 7 6 8 4 3 7 7

CodeBreaker

Use the telephone dial pad and place the correct letter above each number to break the code and solve the

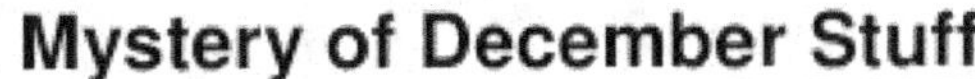

#3 Where the Nobel prize is awarded in December

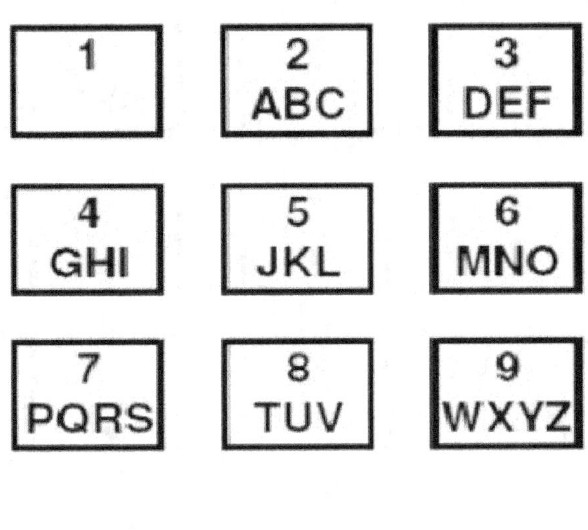

S _ _ _ _ _ _ _ _

7 8 6 3 5 4 6 5 6

#4 Roman holiday celebrated at the end of December

1	2 ABC	3 DEF
4 GHI	5 JKL	6 MNO
7 PQRS	8 TUV	9 WXYZ

S _ _ _ _ _ _ _ _ _

7 2 8 8 7 6 2 5 4 2

CodeBreaker

Use the telephone dial pad and place the correct letter above each number to break the code and solve the

Mystery of December Stuff

#5 Edward VIII married Wallis Warfield Simpson after he did this in December

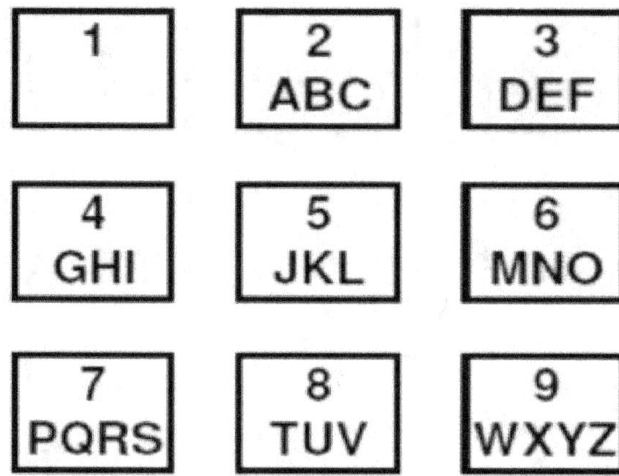

A _ _ _ _ _ _ _ _

2 2 3 4 2 2 8 3 3

#6 You sit on his lap in December

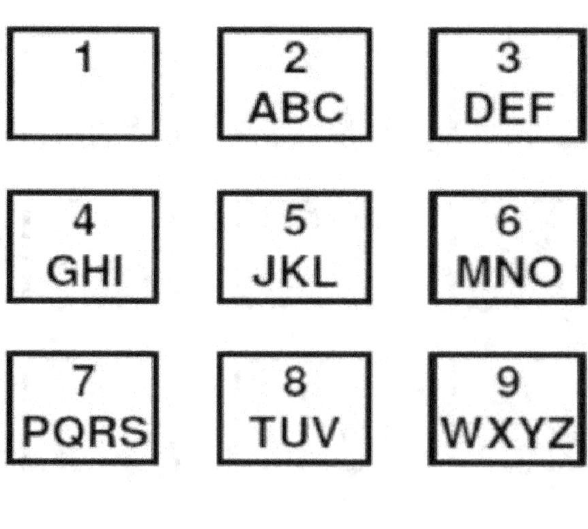

S _ _ _ _

7 2 6 8 2

CodeBreaker

Use the telephone dial pad and place the correct letter above each number to break the code and solve the

More December Mysteries

#1 Born December 25, 1642, this man discovered gravity

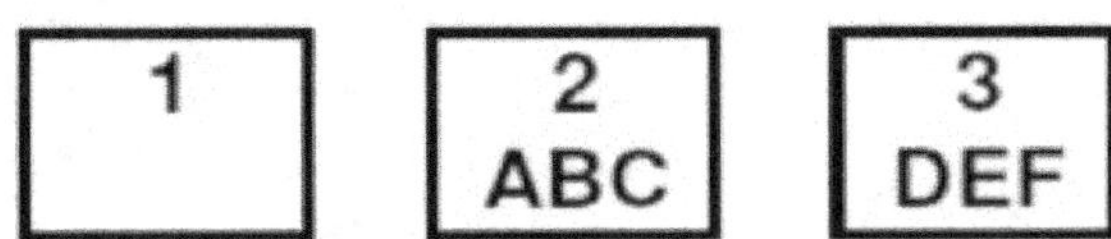

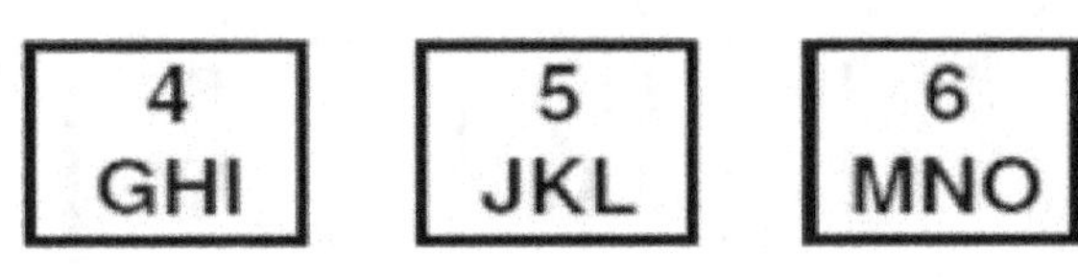

7 PQRS | 8 TUV | 9 WXYZ

S _ _   _ _ _ _ _   _ _ _ _ _ _

7 4 7   4 7 2 2 2   6 3 9 8 6 6

#2 Born December 25, 1821, this woman founded the American Red Cross

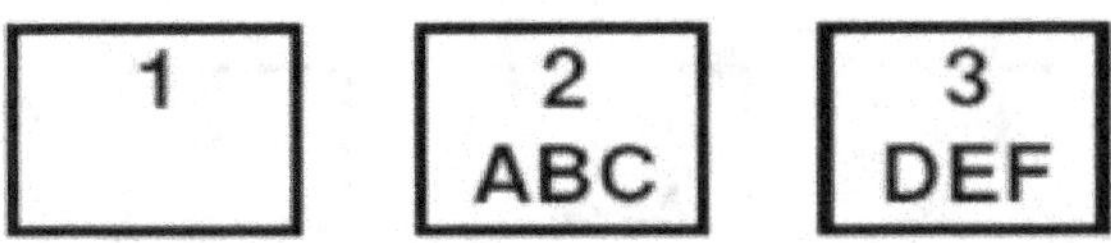

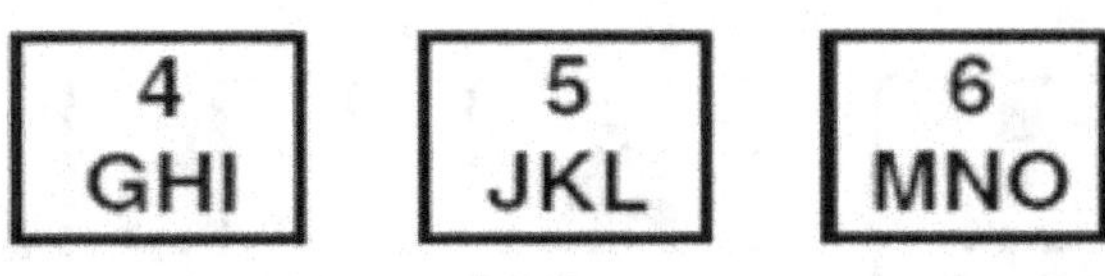

7 PQRS | 8 TUV | 9 WXYZ

C _ _ _ _   _ _ _ _ _ _

2 5 2 7 2   2 2 7 8 6 6

CodeBreaker

Use the telephone dial pad and place the correct letter above each number to break the code and solve the

More December Mysteries

#3 On December 25, 1776, Washington crossed this river to surprise the Hessians

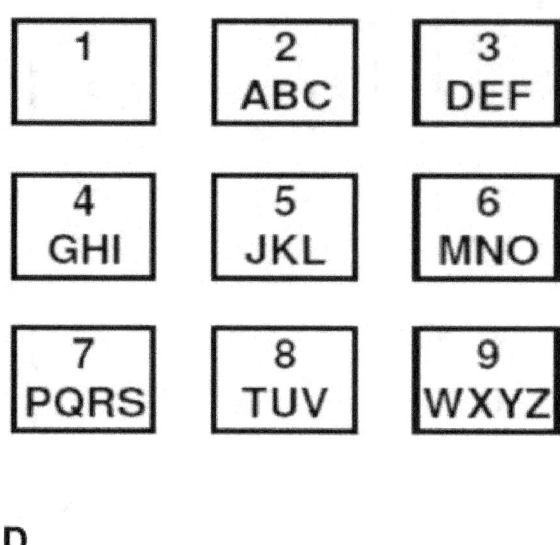

D _ _ _ _ _ _ _

3 3 5 2 9 2 7 3

#4 This little chickadee died on December 25, 1942

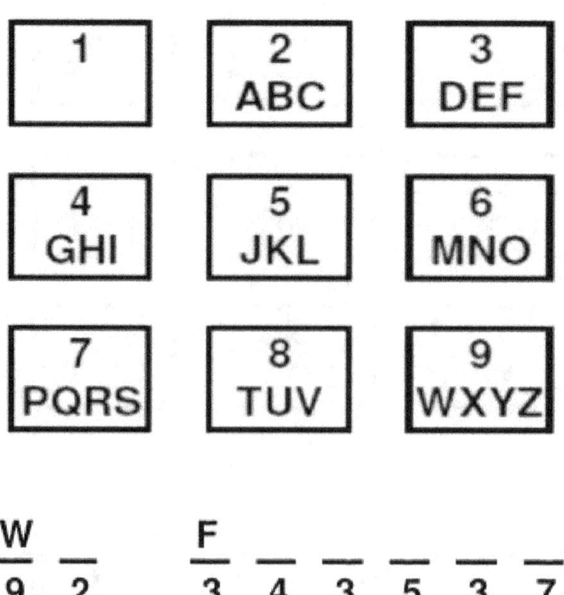

W _ F _ _ _ _ _

9 2 3 4 3 5 3 7

CodeBreaker

Use the telephone dial pad and place the correct letter above each number to break the code and solve the

More December Mysteries

#5 Santa comes down this every December

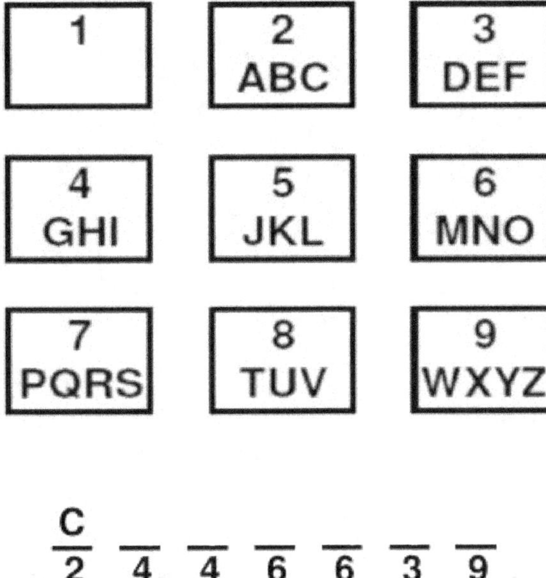

C _ _ _ _ _ _
2 4 4 6 6 3 9

#6 St. Nicholas comes on

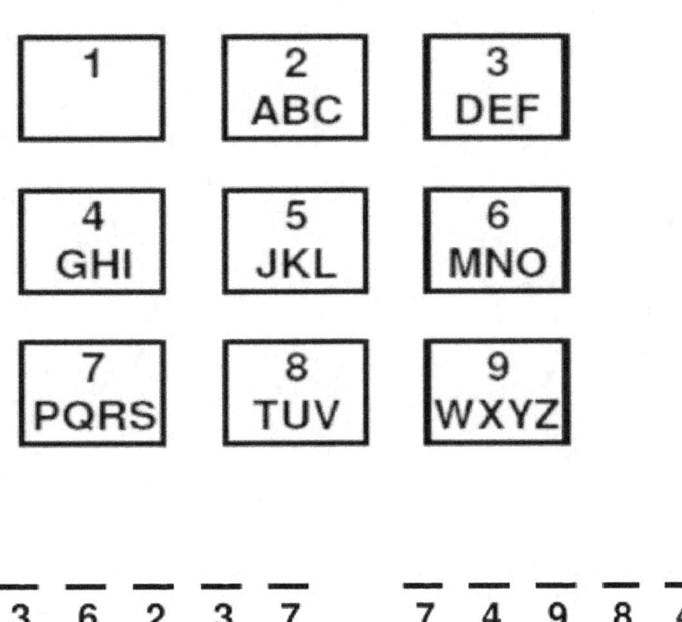

D _ _ _ _ _ _ _   _ _ _ _ _
3 3 2 3 6 2 3 7   7 4 9 8 4

CodeBreaker - Answers

December Mysteries

#1 **W I N T E R   S O L S T A C E**

#2 **M I S T L E T O E**

#3 **W E N C E S L A S**

#4 **F E S T I V A L   O F   L I G H T S**

#5 **P E A R L   H A R B O R**

#6 **G R E G O R I A N**

CodeBreaker - Answers

Awesome December Mysteries

#1 J O E L P O I N S E T T

#2 M I D N I G H T M A S S

#3 I T S A W O N D E R F U L
L I F E

#4 B O S T O N T E A P A R T Y

#5 C H A R L I E C H A P L I N

#6 A C H R I S T M A S S T O R Y

CodeBreaker - Answers

Mystery of December Stuff

#1 F R A N K S I N A T R A

#2 W R I G H T B R O T H E R S

#3 S T O C K H O L M

#4 S A T U R N A L I A

#5 A B D I C A T E D

#6 S A N T A

CodeBreaker - Answers

More December Mysteries

#1 S I R I S A A C N E W T O N

#2 C L A R A B A R T O N

#3 D E L A W A R E

#4 W C F I E L D S

#5 C H I M N E Y

#6 D E C E M B E R S I X T H

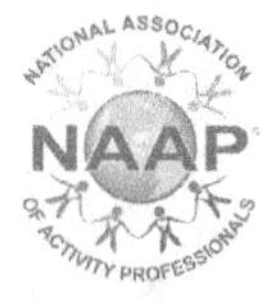

Budget and Time-Saver Activities

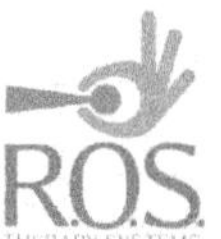

As caregivers, our time and finances can often be strained and stretched to the limit. With that in mind, R.O.S. Therapy Systems has designed activity lesson plans that are easy on the budget and use common household items that are readily available from grocery stores or dollar stores.

Activities are not just playing Bingo. It can be anything! Here are some general activity suggestions that can help you get started and do not cost any money.

Around the House Activities

- Making the bed
- Folding laundry items such as napkins or towels
- Reading the newspaper
- Setting the table
- Watching a favorite television game show or program
- Having a conversation

Please remember that as a caregiver, you should be present at all times. No matter how simple YOU think an activity may be, it may be a challenge for the person you are working with, and they may need assistance or some type of verbal cue. If you have designed an activity on your own or used one of the general suggestions above, please use an Activity Lesson Plan form so that all caregivers may see it. For continuity, they will need to access the notes of any verbal cues or assistance which may have been required or given for the participant to enjoy the activity.

www.ingramcontent.com/pod-product-compliance
Lightning Source LLC
Chambersburg PA
CBHW081223280526
45787CB00006B/2498

9781518604270